BREAST CANCER: PROGRESS IN BIOLOGY, CLINICAL MANAGEMENT AND PREVENTION

DEVELOPMENTS IN ONCOLOGY

Recent Volumes

BREAST CANCER: PROGRESS IN BIOLOGY, CLINICAL MANAGEMENT AND PREVENTION

Proceedings of the International Association for Breast Cancer Research Conference, Tel-Aviv, Israel, March 1989

edited by

Marvin A. Rich
Jean C. Hager
International Association
for Breast Cancer Research
Sint Maarten
Netherlands, Antilles

Iafa Keydar
Tel Aviv University,
Israel

Kluwer Academic Publishers
Boston/Dordrecht/London

Distributors for North America:
Kluwer Academic Publishers
101 Philip Drive
Assinippi Park
Norwell, Massachusetts 02061, USA

Distributors for all other countries:
Kluwer Academic Publishers Group
Distribution Centre
Post Office Box 322
3300 AH Dordrecht, THE NETHERLANDS

Library of Congress Cataloging-in-Publication Data

International Association for Breast Cancer Research. Conference
  (1989 : Tel Aviv, Israel)
    Breast cancer : progress in biology, clinical management, and
  prevention : proceedings of the International Association for Breast
  Cancer Research Conference, Tel-Aviv, Israel, March 1989 / edited by
  Marvin A. Rich, Jean C. Hager, Iafa Keydar.
      p. cm. — (Developments in oncology ; 58)
      ISBN 0-7923-0507-8
      1. Breast—Cancer—Congresses. I. Rich, Marvin A. II. Hager,
  Jean Carol, 1943-   . III. Keydar, Iafa. IV. Title. V. Series.
      [DNLM: 1. Breast Neoplasms—therapy—congresses. 2. Breast
  Neoplasms—prevention—congresses. W1 DE998N v. 58 / WP 870 I578b
  1989]
  RC280.B8154   1989
  616.99 '449—dc20
  DNLM/DLC
  for Library of Congress   89-24432
                                                                  CIP

Printed in the United States of America

CONTENTS

CONTRIBUTORS

I. Ali, National Cancer Institute, Bethesda, MD 20892 USA

Patrick Augereau, Unite Hormones et Cancer, INSERM et
Universite de Montpellier, Montpellier, France

R. W. Baldwin, Cancer Research Campaign Laboratories,
University of Nottingham, Nottingham NG7 2RD, UK

E. W. Blank, John Muir Cancer and Aging Research
Institute, Walnut Creek, CA 94596 USA

Pierre Briozzo, Unite Hormones et Cancer, INSERM et
Universite de Montpellier, Montpellier, France

Jean-Paul Brouillet, Unite Hormones et Cancer, INSERM et
Universite de Montpellier, Montpellier, France

M. Brunet, Centre Rene Huguenin, St Cloud, France

Aman U. Buzdar, University of Texas M.D. Anderson Cancer
Center, Houston, TX USA

R. Cailleau, John Muir Cancer and Aging Research
Institute, Walnut Creek, CA 94596 USA

R. Callahan, National Cancer Institute, Bethesda, MD
20892 USA

Robert D. Cardiff, Department of Pathology, School of
Medicine, University of California, Davis, CA 95616 USA

Francoise Capony, Unite Hormones et Cancer, INSERM et
Universite de Montpellier, Montpellier, France

Vincent Cavailles, Unite Hormones et Cancer, INSERM et
Universite de Montpellier, Montpellier, France

R. L. Ceriani, John Muir Cancer and Aging Research
Institute, Walnut Creek, CA 94596 USA

Pierre Chambon, LGME-CNRS et U184-INSERM, Strasbourg,
France

Ib J. Christensen, University Department of Clinical
Physiology and Nuclear Medicine, The Finsen Institute,
Rigshospitalet, Copenhagen, Denmark

A. J. Clarke, Cancer Research Campaign Laboratories,
University of Nottingham, Nottingham, NG7 2RD, UK

Maria I. Colnaghi, Experimental Oncology E, Instituto Nazionale Tumori, Milano, Italy

E. R. De Sombre, Ben May Institute, Departments of Radiology and Radiation Oncology, The University of Chicago, Chicago IL 60637 USA

Karel A. Dicke, University of Texas M.D. Anderson Cancer Center, Houston, Texas USA

Frank R. Dunphy II, University of Texas M.D. Anderson Cancer Center, Houston, TX USA

Gilles Freiss, Unite Hormones et Cancer, INSERM et Universite de Montpellier, Montpellier, France

H. Galski, Laboratory of Molecular Biology, National Cancer Institute, Bethesda, MD 20892 USA

Marcel Garcia, Unite Hormones et Cancer, INSERM et Universite de Montpellier, Montpellier, France

S. J. Gatley, Ben May Institute, Departments of Radiology and Radiation Oncology, The University of Chicago, Chicago, IL 60637 USA

C. Gautier, LGME-CNRS et U184-INSERM, Strasbourg, France

L. J. Goldstein, Laboratory of Molecular Biology, National Cancer Institute, Bethesda, MD 20892 USA

M. M. Gottesman, Laboratory of Molecular Biology, Bethesda, MD 20892 USA

S. Green, LGME-CNRS et U184-INSERM, Strasbourg, France

N. M. Greenberg, Department of Cell Biology, Baylor College of Medicine, Houston, Texas USA

K. Hacene, Centre Rene Huguenin, St. Cloud, France

Jean C. Hager, International Association for Breast Cancer Research, Simpson Bay, Sint Maarten, Netherlands Antilles

M. Hareuveni, Department of Microbiology, Tel Aviv University, Ramat Aviv, Israel

P. V. Harper, Ben May Institute, Departments of Radiology and Radiation Oncology, The University of Chicago, Chicago, IL 60637 USA

Adrian L. Harris, ICRF Clinical Oncology Unit, Churchill Hospital, Headington, Oxford, OX3 7LJ, England

Pauline Hecht, New York Infirmary-Beekman Downtown Hospital, New York, NY USA

I. Craig Henderson, Dana Farber Cancer Institute, Harvard Medical School, Boston, MA USA

J. Horev, Department of Microbiology, Tel Aviv University, Ramat Aviv, Israel

Gabriel N. Hortobagyi, University of Texas M.D. Anderson Cancer Center, Houston, TX USA

Leonard Horwitz, University of Texas M.D. Anderson Cancer Center, Houston, TX USA

A. Hughes, Ben May Institute Departments of Radiology and Radiation Oncology, The University of Chicago, Chicago, IL 60637 USA

M.-C. Hung, Department of Tumor Biology, University of Texas M.D. Anderson Cancer Center, Houston, TX 77030 USA

Sundar Jagannath, University of Texas M.D. Anderson Cancer Center, Houston, TX USA

J. M. Jeltsch, LGME-CNRS et U184-INSERM, Strasbourg, France

I. Keydar, Department of Microbiology, Tel Aviv University, Ramat Aviv, Israel

M. P. Kieny, Transgene S.A., Strasbourg, France

W. J. King, Ben May Institute Department of Radiology and Radiation Oncology, The University of Chicago, Chicago, IL 60637 USA

Daniel B. Kopans, Department of Radiology, Massachusetts General Hospital and Harvard Medical School, Boston, MA 02114 USA

P. Kotkes, Department of Microbiology, Tel Aviv University, Ramat Aviv, Israel

R. Lathe, LGME-CNRS et U184-INSERM, Strasbourg, France

K.-F. Lee, Department of Cell Biology, Baylor College of Medicine, Houston, TX and Whitehead Institute for Biomedical Research, Cambridge, MA 02142 USA

R. Lidereau, Centre Rene Huguenin, St. Cloud, France

Flora Lubin, Department of Clinical Epidemiology, Chaim Sheba Medical Center, Tel Aviv University Medical School, Tel Hashomer, Israel

Thierry Maudelonde, Unite Hormones et Cancer, INSERM et Universite de Montpellier, Montpellier, France

Baruch Modan, Department of Clinical Epidemiology, Chaim Sheba Medical Center, Tel Aviv University Medical School, Tel Hashomer, Israel

Philippe Montcourrier, Unite Hormones et Cancer, INSERM et Universite de Montpellier, Montpellier, France

I. Pastan, National Cancer Institute, Bethesda, MD 20892 USA

J. S. Peng, John Muir Cancer and Aging Research Institute, Walnut Creek, CA 94596 USA

J. A. Peterson, John Muir Cancer and Aging Research Institute, Walnut Creek, CA 94596 USA

M. R. Price, Cancer Research Campaign Laboratories, University of Nottingham, Nottingham, NG7 2RD, UK

T. V. Reding, Department of Cell Biology, Baylor College of Medicine, Houston, TX USA

Marvin A. Rich, International Association for Breast Cancer Research, Simpson Bay, Sint Maarten, Netherlands Antilles

M. C. Rio, LGME-CNRS et U184-INSERM, Strasbourg, France

Henri Rochefort, Unite Hormones et Cancer, INSERM et Universite de Montpellier, Montpellier, France

Carsten Rose, University Department of Clinical Physiology and Nuclear Medicine, The Finsen Institute, Rigshospitalet, Copenhagen, Denmark

J. M. Rosen, Department of Cell Biology, Baylor College of Medicine, Houston, TX USA

R. Rozin, Tel Aviv Medical Center, Tel Aviv, Israel

I. H. Russo, Department of Pathology, Michigan Cancer Foundation, Detroit, MI 48201 USA

J. Russo, Department of Pathology, Michigan Cancer Foundation, Detroit, MI 48201 USA

J. L. Schwartz, Ben May Institue Departments of Radiology and Radiation Oncology, The University of Chicago, Chicago, IL 60637 USA

N. Smorodinsky, Department of Microbiology, Tel Aviv University, Ramat Aviv, Israel

Jorge A. Spinolo, University of Texas M.D. Anderson Cancer Center, Houston, TX USA

Gary Spitzer, University of Texas M.D. Anderson Cancer Center, Houston TX USA

Robert Strange, Department of Pathology, School of Medicine, University of California, Davis, CA 95616 USA

Susan M. Thorpe, University Department of Clinical Physiology and Nuclear Medicine, The Finsen Institute, Rigshospitalet, Copenhagen, Denmark

C. Tomasetto, LGME-CNRS et U184-INSERM, Strasbourg, France

I. Tsarfaty, Department of Microbiology, Tel Aviv University, Ramat Aviv, Israel

Francoise Vignon, Unite Hormones et Cancer, INSERM et Universite de Montpellier, Montpellier, France

M. Weiss, Department of Microbiology, Tel Aviv University, Ramat Aviv, Israel

M. A. Wong, John Muir Cancer and Aging Research Institute, Walnut Creek, CA 94596 USA

D. H. Wreschner, Department of Microbiology, Tel Aviv University, Ramat Aviv, Israel

Jonathan C. Yau, University of Texas M.D. Anderson Cancer Center, Houston, TX USA

J. Zaretsky, Department of Microbiology, Tel Aviv University, Ramat Aviv, Israel

S. Zrihan, Department of Microbiology, Tel Aviv University, Ramat Aviv, Israel

PREFACE

In breast cancer as in other cancers on the front line of modern interdisciplinary research we have crossed the threshhold of new understanding. Fueled by an awareness that breast cancer is a leading cause of morbidity and mortality in women and honed by rapid technological advances in molecular mechanisms, major inroads into the darkness of this scourge have been accomplished during the past several years.

Basic laboratory and clinical research findings must influence and in turn be influenced by efforts to detect, to diagnose and to cure the human disease. It is indeed gratifying to note that the efforts of scientists and clinicians from throughout the world reported in this volume are achieving this objective.

The first section of the book focuses on the molecular and genetic basis of breast cancer. The role of specific oncogenes in mammary tumorigenesis using transgenic mice and mammary glands correlating molecular events with specific stages in neoplastic development are described and discussed. Such topics as the nature of specific oncogenes, levels of oncogene expression, the alteration of expression of other growth regulatory genes and the state of the cell in which the oncogene is expressed are specifically addressed.

This section of the book is rounded out with discussions on the potential of genetic alterations as indicators of prognosis, the characterization of full-length cDNA codes for breast cancer markers and the function of antigens in tuomorigenesis.

The second group of chapters address a far more pragmatic issue, the state of the art of breast cancer screening, diagnosis, and therapy. A thoughtful evaluation of the survival benefits of local excision, a thorough presentation of perspectives in adjuvant breast cancer chemotherapy past, present, and future, and a look at the genetic basis for the multiple mechanisms of *de novo* or aquired resistance to chemotherapy all contribute to a measured awareness of comparative progress in these vital elements of breast cancer control. This section also provides an important insight into new therapeutic strategies for high dose chemotherapy enabled by autologous bone marrow transplantation.

The chapters in the third section emphasize the ever-shrinking distance between the research laboratory and the breast cancer patient. The role of oral contraceptives in prevention *and* promotion of tumorigenesis reach to the germinal mechanisms and pathogenesis of mammary cancer. Other topics explored in this section include the role of cathepsin-D in diagnosis, prognosis and tumor progression, the relationship between the presence of tumor cells in the bone marrow and specific prognosis, and the development of new approaches to receptor-directed diagnosis and therapy. The last two chapters deal with a much heralded era of hope for the *prevention* of breast cancer through dietary interventions and the development of vaccines.

The battle for the control of breast cancer goes on. Victories are won, new obstacles to true understanding are revealed and sometimes overcome. Many would agree that we are approaching a true molecular understanding of those events we characterize as malignant transformation. We must extend this knowledge to the critical areas of tumor progression and metastasis and to the practical aspects of health behaviour modification aimed at prevention and for those less fortunate, thoughtful and effective therapy.

The results and progress from diverse fields of science and medicine contained in this volume, a report of the biennial research conference of the International Association for Breast Cancer Research held in Tel Aviv in 1989 suggests new areas for exploration, documents critical advances and offers new hope for the conquest of breast cancer. The battle goes on.

Marvin A. Rich
Jean Carol Hager
Iafa Keydar

Sint Maarten, Netherlands Antilles
Tel Aviv, Israel
June, 1989

The editors gratefully acknowledge the support of a grant, CA 50664, from the National Cancer Institute of the United States and the many organizations and individuals whose generous support made the conference and these proceedings possible. We thank Mr. Eric Messier for his patient assistance and valuable technical advice in the preparation of this book.

1

TRANSGENIC MICE AND TRANSGENIC MAMMARY GLANDS

Robert Strange and Robert D. Cardiff

Department of Pathology, School of Medicine, University of California, Davis, CA 95616

INTRODUCTION

Malignant transformation of the mammary gland is a multistep process influenced by many factors, but the relationships between individual factors and specific stages in neoplastic development are not well understood (1-3). Studies utilizing rodent mammary tumor systems have identified activation or expression of oncogenes in mammary tumors, suggesting that these are important factors in mammary tumorigenesis (3,4). However, these studies have not allowed correlation of oncogene expression with specific stages in neoplastic development.

Recently, the development of transgenic animals and transgenic mammary glands has allowed in vivo evaluation of the role of specific oncogenes in mammary tumorigenesis. Expression of oncogenes in transgenic mammary epithelium has confirmed that multiple genetic mutations are required for development of mammary tumors and that oncogenes play important roles in this process. These transgenic mammary systems are now being utilized to correlate expression of specific oncogenes with specific stages in neoplastic development.

Construction of transgenic mice and transgenic mammary glands

Transgenic mice. Transgenic mice are created by introduction of exogenous DNA into the germline of mice. The DNA is injected directly into fertilized mouse eggs. Transgenic mice develop from eggs which incorporate the exogenous DNA. This introduced DNA, or transgene, is potentially carried in all cells and transmitted to progeny in a Mendelian fashion (5).

Transgenic mammary glands. Transgenic mammary glands are constructed by introducing exogenous DNA directly into primary cultures of mammary epithelial cells, usually by infection with retroviral vectors (6,7). The infected epithelial cells are then transplanted into the gland-cleared mammary fat pads of syngenetic mice where they grow to form transgenic mammary outgrowths. Transgenic mammary glands are thus transgenic organs with the exogenous DNA present only in mammary outgrowths of the transplanted epithelial cells.

Transgenic organisms and transgenic organs

The goal of these transgenic systems is similar: to introduce and express exogenous DNA in normal mammary epithelium in a normal growth environment. How do the two systems differ? Overtly stated, one system involves a transgenic organism the other a transgenic organ. Transgenic mice are genetically homogenous, transgenic organisms. Mice in a particular transgenic line carry introduced DNA in the same chromosomal location(s) and transmit it in Mendelian fashion. Thus, it becomes possible to do genetic studies comparing neoplastic influences on mice with the same genetic mutations.

The major limitations of transgenic mice are the need for a tissue specific promoter and the potential for indirect systemic effects due to transgene expression in tissues other than those targeted. In addition, there is selection against mutations that may be important in tumorigenesis but are also embryonic lethals.

In contrast, transgenic mammary glands are genetically heterogenous, transgenic organs. Because introduced oncogenes are introduced only into the target epithelial cells, the potential for unforseen systemic contributions to neoplastic development is minimized. Thus transgenic mammary glands require only that the promoter of an introduced oncogene be functional in mammary epithelium. In addition, because only the mammary gland is effected, mutations that would be lethal during embryonic development also may be evaluated.

The major limitation of transgenic mammary gland systems is the in vitro growth requirement for introducing DNA. Growth of normal cells in vitro has the potential to introduce unforseen changes that could contribute to neoplastic development. However, these changes can be limited by using feeder layer systems or short periods of cell culture (6,7).

NEOPLASTIC DEVELOPMENT IN TRANSGENIC MAMMARY EPITHELIUM

Several oncogenes implicated in development of human mammary tumors have been introduced into transgenic mice but expression of these genes has not resulted in direct malignant transformation of mammary epithelium (8-11). Instead, normal or nonmalignant development of the mammary gland has been observed, followed by development of mammary tumors. Because mammary tumors a ise adjacent to normal mammary tissue that also expresses the introduced oncogene, these experiments support the multistep paradigm for mammary tumorigenesis.

Introduction of oncogenes into transgenic mammary glands has resulted in development of mammary epithelial dysplasias and hyperplasias (6,7). These morphological alterations resemble the premalignant, intermediate stage lesions associated with neoplastic development of the mouse mammary gland (1,2). In the case of myc transgenic mammary glands, this also was accompanied by the development of a mammary tumor (6). Thus, the pattern of mammary neoplasia observed in transgenic mammary glands also is consistent with a multi-stage, neoplastic development.

FACTORS THAT INFLUENCE NEOPLASTIC PROGRESSION

Tumors arise in transgenic mammary epithelium at different rates, implying that interactions between introduced oncogenes and other host factors influence malignant transformation. Experiments using transgenic mammary systems suggest that the factors contributing to malignant transformation include: 1) the particular oncogene expressed, 2) the tissue in which an oncogene is expressed, 3) the level of oncogene expression, 4) the developmental state of the cell in which an oncogene is expressed, 5) alteration of normal cellular growth control stimuli, and 6) mutation or altered expression of other growth control genes. In transgenic mammary epithelium, these factors are controlled by the particular oncogene or combination of oncogenes introduced and the promoter elements used to regulate expression of the oncogenes. The results of oncogene expression and cellular response to that expression are thus reflected in the neoplastic development seen in the transgenic mammary epithelium.

Transgene-associated factors

Tissue specific expression. To study mammary tumorigenesis, an introduced oncogene must be expressed in mammary epithelium. Promoter sequences with tissue specific activities have been utilized to restrict expression of introduced oncogenes to mammary epithelium. The glucocorticoid responsive regulatory elements of the mouse mammary tumor virus long terminal repeat (MMTV LTR) (8) or the lactogenic hormone responsive elements of the whey acidic protein (Wap), a major mouse milk protein, have been used to limit expression of introduced oncogenes to mammary epithelium (9).

MMTV LTR constructs are relatively tissue-specific. High levels of expression are found in mammary epithelium, salivary glands, Harderian glands, and male reproductive organs (10,15). In addition, lower levels of expression are also detected in the brain, thymus, liver, kidney and ovary. Transgenic animals receiving MMTV LTR-regulated oncogenes develop mammary and salivary gland tumors and hyperplasias of the Harderian gland and male reproductive organs (10,12).

The Wap gene promoter confers tissue specificity and hormone-dependent expression onto a Wap-promoted oncogene in transgenic mice. Expression of the whey acidic protein (Wap) is regulated by the lactogenic hormone prolactin, and further modulated by insulin and hydrocortisone levels (14). Expression of Wap chimeric genes is detected only in response to lactogenic stimulus and localized to the mammary gland and, to a lesser degree, the brain of lactating mice (9,11). Wap-promoted oncogenes have resulted in mammary tumors in females. With the exception of one line, males do not express Wap-promoted transgenes or develop tumors (9). Thus, the regulatory sequences directing expression of an oncogene in transgenic mammary epithelium have a significant contribution to neoplastic development. This implies that regulatory sequences of activated oncogenes may play a similar role.

Oncogene expressed. Mammary tumors develop in a random manner, but the particular oncogene expressed in transgenics is also an important determinant in neoplastic development. For example, MMTV/ras transgenics develop Harderian gland hyperplasias but these hyperplasias are not seen in MMTV/myc transgenics (8,10). This does not rule out the presence of myc-induced changes but morphological alterations associated with ras expression suggest that Harderian gland epithelium is more sensitive to activation of a ras oncogene. In contrast, Wap-myc transgenics develop multiple mammary tumors but Wap-ras transgenics only rarely develop mammary tumors (14). Thus, the particular oncogene expressed and tissue in which it is expressed may be important in initiation of neoplastic development.

Level of oncogene expression. Elevated oncogene expression is detected in the mammary tumors of some transgenic lines, but it is not clear whether increased expression is a cause of malignant transformation. For example, the level of transgene expression is much higher in mammary tumors that develop in Wap-promoted transgenics than in the phenotypically normal mammary epithelium that also expresses the oncogene (11). This could be explained by: 1) the greater proportion of epithelial cells in mammary adenocarcinomas than in phenotypically normal mammary glands, 2) the loss of normal hormone sensitivity in the microenvironment of a mammary tumor, or 3) alteration of oncogene DNA in the mammary tumor. However, expression of normal endogenous milk protein genes was not elevated in mammary tumors of a Wap-ras transgenic, indicating that increased expression is not simply a function of a large number of epithelial cells (9). In addition, DNA alterations, suggesting gene amplification or rearrangement, also were not detectable by Southern blot analysis of mammary tumor DNA. In contrast, expression of both the Wap-myc transgene and the normal endogenous whey acidic protein is independent of hormonal status in mammary tumors found in Wap-myc transgenics (11). Thus, elevated expression may involve alteration of oncogene regulatory sequences not detectable by Southern blot analysis or the alteration of expression of other genes involved in regulation of gene expression. These data do suggest that increased expression of an oncogene may contribute to malignant transformation, but the effect appears indirect.

Host Factors

Stages of differentiation and proliferation. The developmental state of the mammary epithelium in which a transgene is expressed also appears to influence tumorigenesis. Expression from a MMTV LTR transgene occurs early in mammary gland development and is enhanced by glucocorticoids. In contrast, Wap-promoted constructs are induced to express when the mammary epithelium, stimulated by lactogenic hormones, is proliferating and undergoing differentiation. MMTV/myc transgenics develop solitary tumors after prolonged latency (8,10). Wap-myc transgenics have a shorter latency, developing tumors in more than one mammary gland and, frequently, multiple tumors in the same mammary gland (11,14). Thus, mammary epithelium stimulated by lactogenic hormones appears to be more susceptible to the influence of the myc oncogene suggesting that the transforming potential of an oncogene can be a function of the differentiated state of the cell as well as the cell type.

Alteration of normal growth stimuli. Alteration of mammary growth control stimuli, such as mediated by hormones, may also contribute to mammary tumorigenesis. One line of MMTV/neu trangenics develops mammary tumors synchronously in all mammary glands with short latency (12). These animals also appear to have hormonal abnormalities. MMTV/neu transgenic females initially show a lactation defect which is followed by the synchronous appearance of mammary tumors. MMTV/neu males develop a hyperplasia of reproductive organs before developing mammary tumors (12). This suggests alteration of the normal hormonal status in both females and males. MMTV/int-1 transgenic males and females both develop mammary hyperplasia prior to developing mammary tumors (13). Curiously, females of these lines also show a lactation defect and males have abnormalities of reproductive organs. Thus, alteration of normal hormonal status may contribute to the rapid malignant progression seen in these animals.

Mutation or activation of additional growth control genes. Mutation of growth control genes appears integral to neoplastic development. The multistep model predicts that malignant progression is dependent upon multiple mutations. Transgenic mice that carry two oncogenes have been constructed by breeding MMTV/myc and MMTV/ras transgenic strains. Although mammary tumors develop randomly from phenotypically normal tissue that expresses both oncogenes, the introduction of two oncogenes is synergistic and results in shorter latency than either oncogene alone (10). Thus, mutation of an additional growth control gene promotes malignant transformation.

A similar rapid development of mammary tumors is seen in transgenic mammary outgrowths of cells infected with HaMSV plus MoMLV (7). The presence of helper virus appears to provide some additional tumorigenic stimulus. This parallels the results of introducing two oncogenes in transgenic mice. The latency is dramatically shortened; tumors have been detected within a month after transplantation in outgrowths of cells infected with both viruses. Mammary dysplasias but no tumors were detected during the period of observation in outgrowths of cells infected with HaMSV alone.

Outgrowths of an established mammary epithelial cell line COMMA-1D are phenotypically similar to premalignant mammary dysplasias, manifesting both cystic ductal structures and a dense lobulo-alveolar hyperplasia (16). Introduction of a Ha-ras oncogene is sufficient to complement the alterations present in COMMA-1D cells and results in rapid development of undifferentiated mammary tumors (14,17). Thus, as predicted by a multistep process, expression of an additional oncogene promotes neoplastic transformation in normal mammary epithelium and promotes malignant progression of premalignant mammary lesions.

Summary

The results of these studies utilizing transgenic mammary systems indicate that expression of a single oncogene in transgenic mammary epithelium does not result directly in malignant transformation but does make the cells more susceptible to subsequent development of tumors. Tumors appear to develop randomly in association with a variety of factors suggesting a stochastic process in which the number of mutations accumulated is more significant than the order of those mutations. The oncogene activated and the interaction of the activated oncogene with other protooncogenes or growth control factors contribute to malignant transformation.

EVALUATION OF A HA-**RAS** ONCOGENE USING A TRANSGENIC MAMMARY GLAND SYSTEM.

We have constructed transgenic mammary glands carrying a viral Ha-ras oncogene to study its role in neoplastic development. These experiments illustrate how a transgenic mammary system can be used to elucidate critical factors in mammary tumorigenesis. We used the Ha-ras oncogene because of its well documented role in mammary cancer (18-25).

Ha-**ras** transgenic mammary glands

For these experiments, cultures of normal mouse mammary epithelial cells were infected using either a genomic clone of the replication-defective HaMSV or wild type HaMSV plus MoMLV helper virus (26-28). The phenotypic effects of expression of the Ha-ras oncogene were evaluated by transplanting the infected cells into surgically-cleared #4 mammary fat pads of BALB/c mice (29). Because the oncogene was introduced only into target cells, it did not require tissue-specific regulatory sequences. The HaMSV LTR, which is functional in mammary epithelium, served as the promoter for the introduced Ha-ras oncogene. Introducing the Ha-ras oncogene only into mammary epithelium also eliminates the potential effects of altered growth stimuli due to expression in other tissues.

Neoplastic development in Ha-**ras** transgenic mammary glands. Twelve weeks after transplantation, the mammary fat pads that received treated mammary epithelial cells were examined. Neoplastic development was seen in outgrowths of cells that received the viral Ha-ras oncogene. Abnormal outgrowths or dysplasias were found in 15/20 outgrowths that developed from cells infected with HaMSV alone; five outgrowths were morphologically normal. Mammary tumors were found in 11/14 outgrowths that developed from cells treated with HaMSV plus helper virus; three outgrowths were dysplastic. All outgrowths that developed from control cells were normal.

Table 1: Types of mammary outgrowths found in transgenic mammary glands.

Treatment	Normal	Dysplasia	Tumor	No Growth	#Fat Pads
Untreated	18	0	0	8	26
HaMSV alone	5	15	0	4	24
HaMSV+MoMLV	0	3	11	14	28
MoMLV alone	7	0	0	17	24
Neomycin^R	7	0	0	3	10

Morphology of transgenic mammary glands

Normal mammary ductal outgrowths resembling host mammary gland developed from untreated cells or control cells (Figure 1: A & B). By contrast,

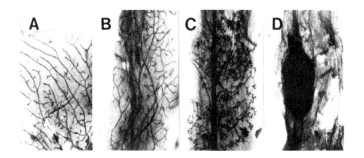

1. Photographs of whole mount preparations of: (A) normal host mammary gland from 4 month-old mouse, (B) a morphologically normal outgrowth that developed from cells infected with a retrovirus carrying a neomycin-resistance gene, (C) dysplastic outgrowth that developed from cells infected with HaMSV alone, and (D) a mammary tumor that developed from cells infected with HaMSV plus a helper virus.

outgrowths of cells infected with HaMSV alone displayed noninvasive, dysplastic features, including enlarged end buds, distended and cystic ducts, and abnormal lobulo-alveolar units (Figure 1: C). Cells infected with both HaMSV and the helper virus rapidly formed mammary tumors (Figure 1: D).

Histology of mammary outgrowths. The histology of the outgrowths of control mammary cells were identical to the orderly, single-layered ducts of the normal host mammary gland (Figure 2: A & B). In contrast, the cells infected with HaMSV alone formed dysplastic outgrowths composed of multi-layered epithelial ducts with poorly organized, enlarged end buds and hyperplastic lobulo-alveolar units (Figure 2: C). These dysplasias were characterized by a high mitotic rate

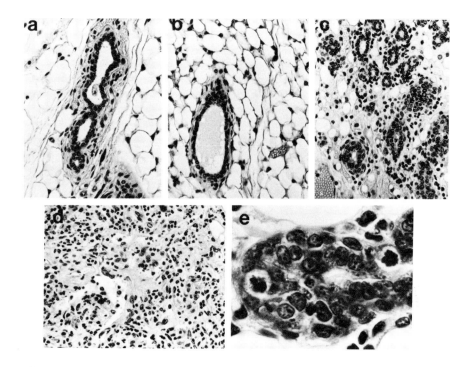

Fig. 2. Photomicrographs of paraffin embedded, hematoxylin and eosin-stained sections of whole mounts demonstrate the histology of: (A) normal host mammary epithelium, (B) an outgrowth of untreated normal mammary epithelial cells, (C) a dysplastic outgrowth that developed from cells infected with HaMSV alone. Contrast the organization of the outgrowths with (D), a poorly-differentiated tumor resulting from treatment of normal mammary epithelial cells with the wild type HaMSV plus the MoMLV helper virus. A high mitotic rate with aberrant cell division was seen in mammary dysplasias as shown at higher magnification in (E).

with a large proportion of abnormal mitoses (Figure 2: E). This abnormal cell division provides a source of mutation required for malignant transformation and is consistent the presence of a population of initiated mammary cells in the dysplasias. Cells treated with HaMSV plus helper virus developed into poorly-differentiated mammary tumors (Figure 2: D).

Detection of the introduced Ha-ras oncogene in mammary neoplasms

Southern blot analysis. Introduction of the viral Ha-ras oncogene into mammary epithelium was confirmed by Southern blot analysis of DNAs from mammary outgrowths and mammary tumors. DNA sequence specific for the introduced viral Ha-ras oncogene was amplified by polymerase chain reaction (7,30). The viral Ha-ras DNA was detected in mammary dysplasias and tumors but not in the normal mammary outgrowths that developed from untreated cells (Figure 3).

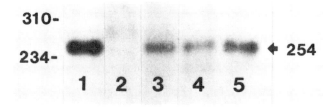

Fig. 3. Southern blot analysis of DNAs, amplified by polymerase chain reaction, from normal and dysplastic mammary outgrowths, a mammary tumor and spleen of animal that received cells infected with HaMSV and MoMLV. DNAs were probed with radiolabelled Ha-ras probe, BS-9. DNAs from: (Lane 1) pBVX vector DNA, (Lane 3) a normal mammary outgrowth of untreated cells, and (Lanes 2 & 4) dysplastic mammary outgrowths of cells infected with HaMSV, (Lane 5) mammary tumor and (Lane 6) spleen of mammary tumor bearing mouse. The arrow indicates the 254 base fragment that is specific for the introduced viral Ha-ras gene. Molecular weight markers are indicated to the left of Lane 1. The amplified vector, tumor and spleen DNAs were diluted 1:250, 1:200 and 1:150 respectively.

Expression of Ha-ras p21. In order to distinguish between expression of the normal cellular Ha-ras gene and the introduced viral Ha-ras oncogene, antisera specific for the viral Ha-ras p21 with a 12th codon arginine mutation was used to identify the viral protein (31). In an immunoblot of ras p21 proteins, expression of the mutated Ha-ras p21 was detected only in mammary dysplasias and mammary tumors or the spleens of animals receiving cells infected with HaMSV plus the helper virus (Figure 4).

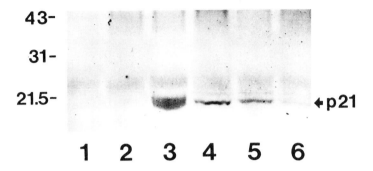

Figure 4.   Immunoblot of immunoprecipitated ras p21 proteins probed with anti-p21-ARG[12] specific antisera (Cetus Corp., Emeryville, CA). Cytoplasmic protein extracts of: (Lane 1) a spleen from an animal receiving mammary cells infected with HaMSV alone, (Lane 2) a pool of normal outgrowths of untreated mammary cells, (Lane 3) a pool of dysplastic outgrowths of mammary cells infected with HaMSV alone, (Lanes 4 & 5) mammary tumors that developed from cells infected with HaMSV plus helper virus and (Lane 6) a spleen from an animal that received mammary cells infected with HaMSV plus helper virus. Molecular weight markers are indicated to the left of lane 1. (Reprinted from reference #7.)

Role of Ha-ras oncogene in mammary dysplasia

Our experiments agree with previous work suggesting that activation of a cellular Ha-ras gene plays a role in mammary neoplasia. Further, these data are consistent with the hypothesis that mutation of a cellular Ha-ras gene can initiate neoplastic development of the mammary gland. Expression of a Ha-ras oncogene into normal mammary epithelial cells appears able to initiate neoplastic development in transgenic mammary glands.

This application of a transgenic mammary gland system has allowed evaluation of the role of a specific oncogene in neoplastic development. The use of a transgenic organ has an advantage over the use of a transgenic organism, ie. a transgenic mouse, for this type of evaluation because it minimizes the potential for unforeseen systemic effects that contribute to malignant transformation but are the result transgene expression in nontarget tissue.

12

SUMMARY

Experiments utilizing transgenic mice have provided new data which are consistent with a multistep model of neoplastic transformation. The introduction of single oncogenes results in random development of mammary tumors, suggestive of a stochastic, random process. The addition of a second oncogene yields tumors with shortened latency period but still in a random manner. In transgenic mice, the systemic effects that result from expression of a transgene in tissues other than the mammary gland, particularly in the brain and reproductive organs, also may contribute to mammary tumorigenesis. The transgenic mammary gland system minimizes such indirect systemic effects.

In similar fashion, introduction oncogenes into transgenic mammary glands has resulted in development of mammary epithelial hyperplasias and dysplasias. These morphological alterations resemble the premalignant, intermediate stage lesions associated with neoplastic development induced by MMTV infection or chemical carcinogenesis (1-3,33). In one case, mammary hyperplasia was accompanied by the development of a mammary tumor (6). In the case of the ras transgenic mammary glands, mammary tumors also developed when a complementing helper virus was present. Thus, the pattern of mammary neoplasia observed in transgenic mammary glands also is consistent with a multi-stage, neoplastic development.

In conclusion, the reconstruction of neoplastic development in transgenic mammary glands and transgenic mice has permitted correlation of molecular events with specific stages in neoplastic development. These systems point to a number of factors that influence malignant transformation, including the particular oncogene or the number of mutated oncogenes, the levels of their expression, the alteration of expression of other growth regulatory genes, and the state of the cell in which an oncogene is expressed. This is just a beginning, as transgenic systems become fully utilized, the interrelations of the various factors implicated in development of cancer will become more clearly understood.

ACKNOWLEDGEMENTS

This work has been supported by grants from the American Cancer Society (CD-235 and MV-428C). R.S. is supported in part by an American Cancer Society Fellowship, California Division, PDB 1-88.

13

REFERENCES

1. Foulds, L. Neoplastic Development, Vol. I, Academic Press, New York, 1969.
2. Cardiff, R.D. Adv. Cancer Res. 42: 167-190, 1984.
3. Morris, D.W. and Cardiff, R.D. Adv. Viral. Oncology 7: 123-140, 1987.
4. Barbacid, M. Ann. Rev. Biochem. 56: 779-827, 1987.
5. Palmiter, R.D. and Brinster, R.L. Ann. Rev. Genet. 20:465-499, 1986.
6. Edwards, P.A.W., Ward, J.L., and Bradbury, J.M. Oncogene 2: 402-412, 1988.
7. Strange, R., Aguilar-Cordova, E., Young, L.J.T., Billy, H., Dandekar, S., and Cardiff, R.D. Oncogene 4: in press, 1989.
8. Stewart, T.A., Pattengale, P.K., and Leder, P., Cell 38: 627-637, 1984.
9. Andres, A.-C., Schönenberger, C.-A., Groner, B., Hennighausen, L., LeMeur, M., and Gerlinger, P. Proc. Natl. Acad. Sci. 84: 1299-1303, 1987.
10. Sinn, E., Muller, W., Pattengale, P., Tepler, I., Wallace, R., and Leder, P. Cell 49: 465-475, 1987.
11. Schönenberger, C.-A., Andres, C.-A., Groner, B., van der Valk, M., LeMeur, M., and Gerlinger, P. EMBO J. 7: 169-175, 1988.
12. Muller, W.J., Sinn,E., Pattengale, P.K., Wallace, R., and Leder, P. Cell 54: 105-115, 1988.
13. Tsukamoto, A.S., Grosschedl, R., Guzman, R., Parslow, T., and Varmus, H.E. Cell 55: 619-625, 1988.
14. Groner, B., Hynes, N.E., Kozma, S., Redmond, S., Saurer, S., Schmitt-Ney, M., Ball, R., Reichman, E., Schönenberger, C., and Andres, A.C. In: Breast Cancer: Cellular and Molecular Biology, (Eds. M.E. Lippmanm and R.B. Dickson), Kluwer Academic Publishers, Boston/Dordrecht/London, 1988, pp. 67-92.
15. Leder, A., Pattengale, P.K., Kuo, A., Stewart, T.A., and Leder, P. Cell 45: 485-495, 1986.
16. Medina, D., Osborn, C.J., Kittrell, F.S., and Ullrich, R.L. J. Natl. Cancer Inst. 76: 1143-1156, 1986.
17. Aguilar-Cordova, E., Strange, R., Young, L.J.T., Billy, H.T., Gumerlock, P. and Cardiff, R.D., manuscript in preparation.
18. Clair, T., Miller, W.R., and Cho-Chung, Y.S. Cancer Res. 47: 5290-5293, 1987.
19. Dandekar, S., Sukumar, S., Zarbl, H., Young, L.J.T., and Cardiff, R.D. Mol. Cell. Biol. 6: 4104-4108, 1986.
20. Horan Hand, P.H., Vilasi, V., Thor, A., Ohuchi, N., and Schlom, J. J. Natl. Cancer Inst. 79: 59-65, 1987.
21. Redmond, S.M.S., Reichman, E., Muller, R., Friis,R.R., Groner, B., and Hynes, N. Oncogene 2: 259-265, 1988.
22. Tanaka, T., Slamon, D.J., Battifora, H., and Cline, M.J. Cancer Res. 46: 1465-1470, 1986.
23. Zarbl, H., Sukumar, S., Arthur, A.V., Martin-Zanca, M., and Barbacid, M. Nature 315: 382-385, 1985.
24. Yokota, J., Tsunetsugu-Yokota, Battifora, H., Le Fevre, C., and Cline, M.J. Science 231: 261-265, 1986.
25. Kraus, M.H., Yuasa, Y., and Aaronson, S.A. Proc. Natl. Acad. Sci. USA 81: 5384-5388, 1984.
26. Ehmann, U.K., Peterson, W.D., and Misfeldt, D.S. J. Cell Biol. 98: 1026-1032, 1984.

14

27. Ellis, R.W., De Feo, D., Maryak, J.M., Young, H.A., Shih, T.Y., Chang, E.H., Lowy, D.R., and Scolnick, E.M. J. Virology 36: 408-420, 1980.
28. Hager, G.L., Chang, E.H., Chan, H.W., Garon, C.F., Israel, M.A., Martin, M.A., Scolnick, E.M., and Lowy, D.R. J. Virol. 31: 795-809, 1979.
29. Ehmann, U.K., Guzman, R.C., Osborn, R.C., Young, L.J.T., Cardiff, R.D., and Nandi, S. J. Natl. Cancer Inst. 78: 751-757, 1987.
30. Saiki, R.K., Gelfand, D.H., Stoffel, S., Scharf, S.J., Higuchi, R., Horn, G.T., Mullis, K.B., and Erlich, H.A. Science 239: 487-491, 1988.
31. Wong, G., Arnheim, N., Clark, R., McCabe, P., Innis, M., Aldwin, L., Nitecki, D., and McCormick, F. Cancer Res. 46: 6029-6033, 1986.
32. Medina, D. In: The mouse in biomedical research, Vol. IV. Experimental biology and oncology (Eds. H.L. Foster, J.D. Small and J.G. Fox), Academic Press, New York, 1982, pp. 373-396.
33. Ethier, S.P., Adams, L.M., and Ullrich, R.L. Cancer Res. 44: 4517-4522, 1984.

2

THE REGULATION OF TISSUE-SPECIFIC CASEIN GENE EXPRESSION IN TRANSGENIC ANIMALS

N. M. GREENBERG[1], T.V. REDING[1], K.-F. LEE[1]*, M.-C. HUNG[2], AND J.M. ROSEN[1]

[1]Department of Cell Biology, Baylor College of Medicine, One Baylor Plaza, Houston, Texas USA, [2]Department of Tumor Biology, The University of Texas System Cancer Center, M.D. Anderson Hospitsal and Tumor Institute, 1515 Holcombe Blvd., Houston, Texas, 77030. *Present address: Whitehead Institute for Biomedical Research, 9 Cambridge Center, Cambridge, Massachusetts, 02142

INTRODUCTION

Multiple factors are known to influence the expression of the caseins, the predominant milk proteins. The caseins are encoded by a small gene family present as a gene cluster on mouse chromosome 5 (1,2). Expressed in a tissue- and stage-specific manner, casein gene expression is also regulated by peptide and steroid hormones (3,4) as well as cell-cell and cell-substratum interactions. (5,6). The ß-casein gene is the most well characterized member of this gene family and is expressed as the predominant milk protein mRNA by the eighth day of lactation when it accounts for approximately 20% of poly(A)+ mRNA (7,8). We have, therefore, chosen to study the molecular mechanisms involved in regulating ß-casein gene expression.

The ability to introduce foreign DNA into the germ line of mice by microinjection into fertilized eggs yielding lines of transgenic mice has facilitated our investigation of the cis-acting elements regulating ß-casein gene expression. Initially, lines of transgenic mice were established carrying an entire rat ß-casein genomic DNA fragment (9). This ß-casein transgene was expressed in a tissue-specific and developmentally-regulated fashion in several independent lines of mice. In subsequent experiments, transgenes were specifically designed to delimit the minimal genetic elements required for directing tissue-specific and hormonally-regulated gene expression. In these experiments, various ß-casein 5' flanking DNA fragments were used to drive a bacterial chloramphenicol acetyltransferase (CAT) reporter gene (10). Using two ß-casein CAT fusion genes driven by either 2.3 kb or 0.5 kb of 5' flanking DNA and containing the non-coding exon I and a portion of intron A, CAT activity was targeted predominately to the mammary gland of transgenic mice. As with the entire ß-casein transgene, both fusion transgenes were expressed in a tissue-specific and developmentally appropriate fashion. However, the absolute levels of expression of the entire ß-casein gene and both fusion genes were only 1% or less of those found for the endogenous ß-casein gene. One current project in our laboratory is the optimization of a ß-casein derived expression vector for targeting expression of heterologous functional genes to the mammary gland in transgenic mice. This optimized vector should have important applications in biotechnology and should also be a valuable tool in the study of normal mammary gland development and tumorigenesis in transgenic animals.

The development of an inducible, tissue-specific expression vector will also facilitate the study of the role of oncogene expression in mammary tumorigenesis. The neu (c-erbB-2) oncogene has been implicated in the development of human breast cancer. A high percentage of human breast cancers have been found to contain amplified copies of the neu gene and many of these tumors also show a high level of neu protein expression (11,12). It has also been reported that there is a correlation between the amplification of neu and relapse and survival in breast cancer patients (13,14). To investigate how the level and timing of neu expression affect normal mammary development and carcinogenesis, the ß-casein based expression vector system has been employed to express the rat neu oncogene in transgenic mice.

MATERIALS AND METHODS

Enzymes and plasmids

Restriction enzymes and DNA modifying enzymes were purchased from Bethesda Research Laboratories and Boehringer Mannheim. All enzymes were used according to the manufacturers' specifications. The isolation of the entire rat ß-casein gene and construction of the 2.3 kb and 0.5 kb 5' flanking ß-casein CAT fusion transgenes has been described previously (9,10,15). The following strategy was used to generate an enhanced ß-casein construct: a mouse mammary tumor virus long terminal repeat (MMTV) Hinf1 cleaved DNA fragment (-428 to -69) containing four glucocorticoid response elements (GRE) was obtained in the Xba1 site of the pBLCAT2 vector (pBLCAT2-GRE) as a gift from M. Parker (Imperial Cancer Research Fund Laboratories, London). Following restriction of pBLCAT2-GRE with BamH1 the resulting 5' overhang ends were converted to blunt ends with Klenow in the presence of all four dNTPs and synthetic HindIII linkers (New England BioLabs) were attached. The GRE fragment was then liberated as a 408 bp HindIII cartridge and purified by a low-melting agarose procedure (16). The purified GRE fragment was inserted in its correct orientation into the unique HindIII site 330 bp upstream of ß-casein exon I in the -524/+490 CAT fusion gene creating the GRE construct. The entire GRE containing construct was liberated as an Nde1-BamH1 fragment, purified by a low-melting agarose procedure and recovered by GeneClean (Bio101) for microinjection.

Constructs bearing the ß-casein neu oncogene cDNA fusion genes were assembled in the pGEM4 vector (Promega). The ß-casein -524/+490 Xbal cartridge was inserted into the Xbal site and the SV40t and poly(A) fragment of pSVoCAT (10) was inserted into the HincII site. Following digestion with Sal1 and subsequent conversion to blunt ends with Klenow and dNTPs the 4.7 kb neuN and neuT cDNAs were individually inserted as blunt ended fragments. The two ß-casein-neu fusion construct genes were excised by SphI and KpnI digestion and purified by a low-melting agarose procedure (16) and recovered by GeneClean (Bio101) for microinjection.

Generation and screening of transgenic mice

Transgenic mice were generated and mouse tail DNA was isolated as described previously (9,10). GRE constructs were screened by polymerase chain reaction (PCR) with 25mer oligonucleotide primers corresponding to the 3' terminal region of the ß-casein fragment and the 5' terminal region of the SV40 fragment. All PCR reactions were performed for 30 cycles in a Perkin Elmer DNA Thermocycler with each cycle being 1 min at 94°, 2 min at 60° and 3 min at 72°. Each reaction contained 1 µg of tail DNA and 2.5 units of AmpliTaq polymerase (Cetus). PCR products were analyzed on 1% agarose gels cast and run in 0.5X TBE buffer (16) and visualized by ethidium bromide staining. Positive neuN and neuT transgenic mice were identified by BamH1 digestion of 10 µg tail DNA and subsequent Southern blotting (16). A random-primed 800 bp BamH1 fragment was used as probe. Transgene copy numbers were determined by DNA slot-blots (9,10) with several inputs of plasmid DNA as titrated standards.

CAT assays

Tissue extracts were prepared by homogenization as described previously (10). Initially 100 µg of protein were used in CAT activity assays with approximately 250 nCi of ^{14}C-chloramphenicol (Amersham, specific activity 57 mCi/mmol). All assays were performed for 2 hr incubations at 37° and optimized with decreasing amounts of protein. Following chromatography using silica gel TLC sheets (Baker), development in chloroform:methanol (95:5) and autoradiography, acetylated and unacetylated forms were excised and quantitated by liquid scintillation spectrometry. After background subtraction of signals observed with tissues of non-transgenic mice the results were expressed as pmol ^{14}C chloramphenicol converted per hr per µg protein.

RESULTS AND DISCUSSION

<u>GRE enhanced expression of ß-casein vectors</u>

Independent lines of transgenic mice have been previously established carrying the entire rat ß-casein gene and two ß-casein CAT fusion genes as illustrated in Fig. 1. In these lines the levels of transgene expression were only 1% or less of the endogenous ß-casein gene, even though the constructs contained sufficient genetic information to target transgene expression to mammary tissue in a developmentally-regulated fashion (9,10). These findings, together with the existence of the caseins as a gene cluster on mouse chromosome 5, suggested that these constructs were perhaps missing enhancer elements required for the appropriate coordinated expression of the caseins in a mammary tissue-specific fashion. Since the enhancer elements for other mammalian genes have been found quite far, e.g. up to 50 kb, 5'- or 3'- from their cognate genes (17,18), and a mammary specific enhancer element has yet to be identified, we have chosen to incorporate the well characterized GRE enhancer derived from the MMTV LTR in our ß-casein driven expression system. This enhancer contains four consensus

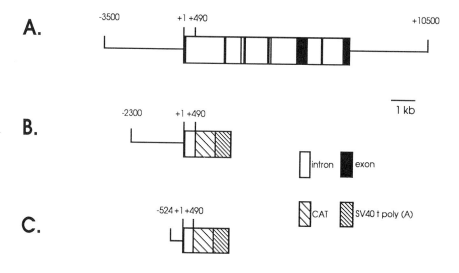

FIGURE 1. Schematic representation of the ß-casein transgenes. A, the entire 14 kb rat genomic ß-casein gene; B, the CAT fusion transgene with 2.3 kb of ß-casein 5' flanking DNA; C, the CAT fusion transgene with 0.5 kb of ß-casein 5' flanking DNA. The first base of ß-casein Exon I is numbered +1.

A. STRUCTURE OF THE RAT ß-CASEIN DIRECTED CAT TRANSGENE

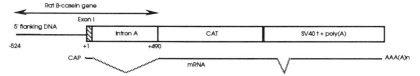

B. STRUCTURE OF THE GRE ENHANCED RAT ß-CASEIN DIRECTED CAT TRANSGENE

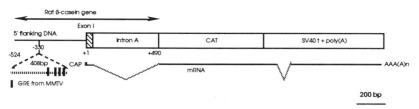

FIGURE 2. Construction of the GRE enhanced -524/+490 ß-casein CAT fusion gene. The 408 bp MMTV LTR DNA fragment containing the four GRE elements as a HindIII cassette (see Materials and Methods) was inserted into the unique HindIII site 330 bp upstream of ß-casein Exon I in the -524/+490 vector (A) yielding the GRE construct (B). The expected mRNA transcript CAP and splice sites are shown.

glucocorticoid response elements and has been demonstrated previously to be both active and hormonally regulated in mammary tissue in transgenic mice (19,20).

As shown in Fig. 2, the MMTV derived GRE was inserted into the unique HindIII site 330 bp upstream of the ß-casein CAP site. This site was chosen because it should not interrupt important β-casein promoter functional elements; it is upstream of the most highly conserved region of the β-casein promoter (21), and is 5' to the region shown to be important for hormonal induction in cell transfection experiments(3,22). The GRE construct was isolated, microinjected into pronuclei of fertilized embryos and ten independent lines of transgenic mice were established. The six female founder mice were mated with non-transgenic males. Male founder mice were bred with non-transgenic females and transgenic female progeny were subsequently mated to non-transgenic males. On the tenth day of lactation one of the fourth mammary glands was biopsied from each mouse under anesthesia and tissue extracts prepared as described

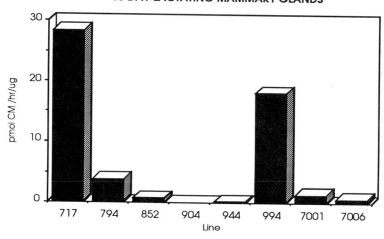

**COMPARISON OF GRE ENHANCED CAT ACTIVITY IN
10 DAY LACTATING MAMMARY GLANDS**

FIGURE 3. Comparison of GRE enhanced CAT activitiy in 10 day lactating mammary glands. To determine whether the GRE would enhance ß-casein CAT gene expression in transgenic mice, mammary glands were biopsied from eight transgenic female animals at 10 days of lactation and the tissues were assayed for CAT activity as described in materials and methods. The activity is reported in pmol of chloramphenicol (CM) converted to acetylated forms per hr per µg protein.

(10). As is shown in Fig.3, of the GRE lines found to express CAT, activities ranged from 0.1 to 28 pmol/ hr/µg protein with an average of 7.6 pmol/hr/µg . The highest expressing line designated #717, expressed at a level significantly greater than any of our fusion lines without the GRE (data not shown). This line was investigated further in order to determine the tissue distribution of CAT expression. Approximately 4-fold more CAT activity was found in the mammary gland than in the thymus, which was the next highest expressing tissue (Fig. 4). Interestingly, thymic expression had been observed previously in our other lines of mice bearing ß-casein driven transgenes (Fig. 1B,C) which did not contain the GRE (9,10).

We have detected CAT expression in the mammary glands of all our expressing lines of transgenic mice carrying ß-casein driven constructs. In the lines carrying the -524/+490 ß-casein CAT fusion genes (Fig. 1C) we had detected expression in the thymus but not in the intestine, brain or salivary gland. However, the enhanced expression of this construct conferred by the GRE may have raised the CAT activity in these tissues to a level now detectable in our assay (Fig. 4). It is also interesting to note that the expression of CAT activity does not necessarily reflect the distribution of glucocorticoid receptors in these

TISSUE DISTRIBUTION IN LINE 717 OF
GRE ENHANCED ß-CASEIN DIRECTED CAT ACTIVITY

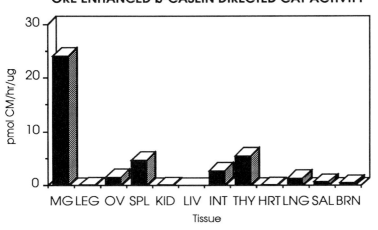

FIGURE 4. Tissue distribution in line 717 of GRE enhanced ß-casein directed CAT activity. An F₁ female of founder GRE mouse 717 was sacrificed at 10 days of lactation and tissues were assayed for CAT activity. MG, mammary gland; LEG, leg muscle; OV, ovary, oviduct and uterus; SPL, spleen; KID, kidney; LIV, liver; INT, intestine; THY, thymus; HRT, heart; LNG, lung; SAL, salivary gland; BRN, brain. Activity is expressed in pmol chloramphenicol (CM) converted to acetylated forms per hr per µg protein.

tissues. In addition, as shown in Fig. 3, not all GRE lines display high levels of CAT expression. This may in part be due to the variability in the site of integration of the transgene.

While an absolute tissue preference for the mammary gland has not been maintained in all GRE lines, it can be generally concluded that in mice carrying the GRE construct, a greater percentage express CAT activity in the mammary gland, and the average level of expression is higher than in our -524/+490 lines lacking the GRE. These experiments have shown the applicability of using a heterologous enhancer to increase the expression of our ß-casein driven constructs and maintain tissue preference for the mammary gland. This is an especially useful approach for transgenic systems in which the cognate enhancer elements have yet to be identified or characterized for a particular promoter. An important consideration in these experiments is the mechanism by which the heterologous enhancer increases expression from a tissue-specific, developmentally-regulated promoter. For example, experiments are currently underway to determine whether the GRE transgene is initiating transcription at the authentic ß-casein start site, in a manner analogous to the parental ß-casein gene, and whether GRE enhanced expression is developmentally regulated and glucocorticoid inducible. These experiments will be of particular interest since tissue-specific promoters, in some cases, act independently with heterologous enhancers (23) while in other instances, increased expression is only observed with the cognate enhancers (24,25,26).

ß-casein neu transgenic mice

For this meeting on mammary cancer we wanted to present some preliminary results of our studies targeting the neu oncogene to the mammary glands of transgenic mice with ß-casein driven constructs. To investigate how the level and timing of neu oncogene expression effects normal mammary development and carcinogenesis, we have established lines of transgenic mice carrying the ß-casein neuN and ß-casein neuT oncogenes (Fig. 5). The activated neuT gene was identified from mRNA of an ethylnitrosourea-induced rat neuroblastoma (27) and the only difference between the genes is a single base point mutation altering a valine residue (neuN) to a glutamic acid residue (neuT) in the predicted transmembrane coding domain (28). Transgenic founder animals were identified by Southern blots using 10 µg of BamH1 digested tail DNA hybridized with a BamH1 fragment of neu cDNA (as shown in Fig. 6). Both a 10 kb band which results from restriction of the endogenous c-neu gene (Fig. 6, lane A) as well as the 0.8 kb fragment which is derived from the transgene (Fig. 6, lane B) were identified.

STRUCTURE OF THE RAT ß-CASEIN neu ONCOGENES

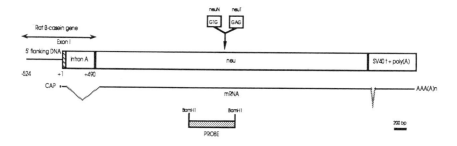

FIGURE 5. Representation of the ß-casein neu transgenes. The 4.7 kb cDNA for either neuN or neuT was fused to the -524/+490 ß-casein cassette. The neuN and neuT cDNAs differ only at a single base in the transmembrane encoding portion of the oncogene. Mice were screened by probing with the 0.8 kb BamH1 fragment shown as a closed box beneath the neu gene. The expected mRNA transcript CAP and splice sites are shown.

A B C D E F G H I J K L M

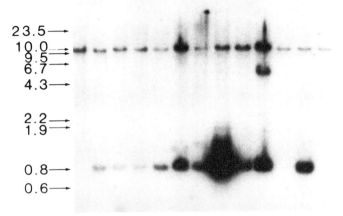

FIGURE 6. Screening for mice carrying the ß-casein neuN and neuT transgenes. Genomic DNA from tail resections was restricted with BamH1, fractionated on a 1% agarose gel, transferred to nitrocellulose membrane, hybridized with a ^{32}P labelled BamH1 probe fragment (see Fig.5) and exposed to X-ray film. The resulting autoradiogram reveals the presence of the 10 kb fragment of the endogenous neu gene as well as the 0.8 kb fragment derived from the transgenes. Sizes in kb are shown on the left. Lane A, non-transgenic mouse DNA; B, non-transgenic mouse with one-copy equivalent of 0.8kb insert; C-I, mice injected with ß-casein neuT; J-M, mice injected with ß-casein neuN .

Independent lines of mice have been identified which carry variable copy numbers ranging from one copy (Fig. 6, lane C) to approximately 50 copies (Fig. 6, lane H) of the ß-casein neu transgenes.

Initially, six independent lines of neuT mice have been generated, of which five have transmitted the transgene to their offspring in a Mendelian fashion. One founder female, number 6448 is now over a year old. We have bred the 6448 founder (Fig. 7) and inbred first generation transgenic offspring to generate homozygous transgenic mice. The 6448 founder female has yet to display any palpable mammary tumors after three litters, even though the ß-casein promoter is maximally induced during lactation in response to lactogenic hormones. Analysis of mammary gland whole mounts following regression (at least five weeks post weaning) also has failed to detect mammary hyperplasia in this line. To determine whether the transgene is being expressed, total RNA from lactating mammary tissues of line 6448 as well as other neuN and neuT lines has been analyzed by Northern blotting. Only very low levels of neu mRNA (at the limit of sensitivity of these blots) have been detected in 20 µg of poly (A)+ selected mRNA (results not shown). Further studies utilising the more sensitive PCR and RNase mapping

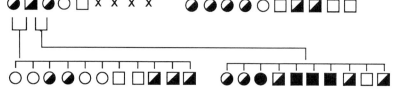

PEDIGREE FOR neuT TRANSGENIC MOUSE 6448

FIGURE 7. Pedigree showing the inheritance of the ß-casein neuT transgene. Transgenic founder female number 6448 carrying the ß-casein neuT transgene was mated with a non-transgenic male and resulting offspring were screened for presence of the transgene by Southern blotting. Of the offspring heterozygous for the transgene, two littermates were subsequently mated yielding a number of homozygous transgenic mice.

techniques will be needed to accurately determine the level and time of onset of transgene expression.

The ß-casein promoter fragment used in our constructs has been shown to direct expression at levels well below those of the endogenous ß-casein gene (see above). This low level of transgene expression in the ß-casein neu mice may explain the absence of a visible neoplastic phenotype in these lines. In studies carried out with MMTV neuT constructs, several independent lines of transgenic mice which expressed significant levels of neuT mRNA in mammary epithelium developed mammary carcinomas (29). In the MMTV neuT mice, the tumors arose in a synchronous fashion, were independent of the number of pregnancies and litter size, and apparently did so through a single-step action of the neuT oncogene (29). The c-myc and v-Ha-ras oncogenes also have been expressed under the control of the MMTV promoter in transgenic mice (30). In mice individually expressing the MMTV c-myc or MMTV v-Ha-ras constructs, the transgenes were found to be expressed in the female mammary gland and caused malignant transformation. However, when both constructs were coexpressed following mating in the F1 animals the kinetics of tumor formation in these animals showed a synerginistic effect with respect to enhanced penetrance and decreased mean survival time (30). In contrast to the results with MMTV driven constructs, when c-myc and v-Ha-ras were targeted to the mammary gland by the whey acidic protein (Wap, another milk protein) promoter, tumors arose in expressing tissues only after long latency periods and several pregnancies and there was no synergism observed for animals coexpressing the two transgenes (31). It is interesting to note that endogenous Wap is expressed at a lower level than ß-casein in non-lactating tissue and Wap is induced later than ß-casein in mammary development. These observations suggest that the promoter-dependent timing and level of oncogene expression during development are important parameters in the transformation of the target tissue. Therefore, a vector permitting low level neu expression directed by a mammary specific promoter might be advantageous for studying the role and timing of neu expression on normal mammary development. Mice carrying such a transgene might also be used to investigate the combined effects of exposing low-level neu expressing mice to limited amounts of carcinogens of either chemical or environmental origin, or the effects of mating such mice to those over-expressing growth hormone. Enhancement of the ß-casein neu constructs with the GRE element of MMTV may prove more useful in future studies since oncogene expression was observed to be enhanced in the malignant tissues of the MMTV neuT mice (29).

There is evidence in the literature which suggests that introns increase transcriptional efficiency in transgenic mice and that this effect is particularily pronounced on genes exposed to developmental influences (32). The vector used in our constructions utilizes a ß-casein intron A 5' splice donor and a putative cryptic 3' acceptor as well as a small splice in the SV40 t segment of the transgene (Fig. 5). These splice sites and the very large exon size, may therefore not be optimal for achieving maximal transgene expression efficiency. As an alternative, genomic neu DNA is being employed in future constructs. Thus, by combining the advantage of the GRE enhanced ß-casein promoter with genomic neu DNA, we should better be able to study the role of timing and extent of oncogene expression on transformation in transgenic mice.

CONCLUSIONS

Having established lines of transgenic mice carrying an entire rat ß-casein genomic DNA fragment and ß-casein CAT fusion genes, we have begun to delimit the cis-acting ß-casein elements required for directing tissue-specific and hormonally-regulated gene expression. The low levels of transgene expression observed in transgenic mice, compared to that of endogenous ß-casein, indicated that the constructs used in these studies lack mammary-specific enhancer elements. By introducing the MMTV GRE into the 5' flanking region of ß-casein, expression of these vectors was enhanced, and as observed in our previous lines, tissue-specificity was not strictly maintained.

Lines of mice carrying ß-casein- neuN and neuT fusion genes have been established.

These transgenes were expressed at very low levels, which may explain why year-old female founder mice have yet to display palpable tumors even after three pregnancies. Over-expression of the ß-casein neu fusion genes with the MMTV GRE, may facilitate our investigation of how the level and timing of neu expression effects normal mammary development and carcinogenesis.

REFERENCES

1. Gupta, P., D'Eustachio, P., Ruddle, F.H., and Rosen, J.R. J. Cell Biol. 93:199-204, 1982
2. Geissler, E.N., Cheng, S.V., Gueslla, J.F., and Housman, D. Proc. Natl. Acad. Sci. 85:9635-9639, 1988
3. Rosen, J.M., Rodgers, J.R., Couch, C.H., Bisbee, C.A., David-Inouye, Y., Campbell, S.M., and Yu-Lee, L.-Y. Anal. N.Y. Acad. Sci 478:63-76, 1986
4. Rosen, J.R., Matusik, R.J., Richards, D.A., Gupta, P., and Rodgers, J.R. Recent Prog. Horm. Res. 36:157-194, 1980
5. Eisenstein, R.S., and Rosen, J.M. Mol. Cell. Biol. 8:3183-3190, 1988
6. Levine, J.F., and Stockdale, F.E. J. Cell Biol. 100:1415-1422, 1985
7. Rosen, J.M., Woo, S.L.C., and Comstock, J.P. Biochem. 14:2895-2903, 1975
8. Hobbs, A.A., Richards, D.A., Kessler, D.J., and Rosen, J.M. J. Biol. Chem. 257:3598-3605, 1982
9. Lee, K.-F., DeMayo, F.J., Atiee, S.H., and Rosen, J.M. Nucl. Acids Res. 16:1027-10412, 1988
10. Lee, K.-F., Atiee, S.H., and Rosen, J.M. Mol. Cell. Biol. 9:560-565, 1989
11. Kraus, M.H., Popescu, N.C., Amsbaugh, S.C., and King, C.R. EMBO J. 6:605-610, 1987
12. van de Vijver, M., van de Bersselaar, R., Devilee, P., Cornalisse, C., Peterse, J., and Nusse, R. Mol. Cell. Biol. 7:2019-2023, 1987
13. Ali, I.U., Campbell, G., Lidereau, R., and Callahan, R. Science 240:1795-1796, 1988
14. Slamon, D.J., and Clark, G.M. Science 240:1796-1798, 1988
15. Jones, W.K., Yu-Lee, L.-Y., Clift, S.M., Brown, T.L., and Rosen, J.M. J. Biol. Chem. 260:7042-7050, 1985
16. Maniatis, T., Fritsch, E.F., and Sambrook, J. Molecular cloning: a laboratory manual. Cold Spring Harbour, 1982
17. Grosveld, F., van Assendelft, G.B., Greaves, D.R., and Kollias, G. Cell 51:975-985, 1987
18. Donoghue, M., Ernst, H., Wentworth, B., Nadal-Ginard, B., and Rosenthal, N. Genes Develop. 2:1779-1790, 1988
19. Ross, S.R., and Solter, D. Proc. Natl. Acad. Sci. USA 82:5880-5884, 1985
20. Stewart, T.A., Hollingshead, P.G., and Pitts, S.L. Moll. Cell. Biol. 8:473-479, 1988
21. Yu-Lee, L.-Y., Richter-Mann, L., Couch, C.H., Stewart, A.F., Mckinlay, A.C., and Rosen, J.M. Nucl. Acids Res. 14:1883-1902, 1987
22. Doppler, W., Groner, B., and Ball, R.K., Proc. Natl. Acad. Sci. USA 86:104-108, 1989
23. Ornitz, D.M., Hammer, R.E., Davison, B.L., Brinster, R.L., and Palmiter, R.D. Mol. Cell. Biol. 7:3466-3472, 1987
24. Pinkert, C.A., Ornitz, D.M., Brinster, R.L., and Palmiter, R.D. Genes and Develop. 1:268-276, 1987
25. Behringer, R.R., Hammer, R.E., Brinster, R.L., Palmiter, R.D., and Townes, T.M. Proc. Natl. Acad. Sci. USA 84:7056-7060, 1987
26. Kollias, G., Hurst, J., deBoer, E., and Grosveld, F. Nucl. Acids Res. 15:5739-5747, 1987
27. Schechter, A.L., Stern, D.F., Vaidyanathan, L., Decker, S.J., Drebin, J.A., Greene, M.I. and Weinberg, R.A. Nature (London) 312:513-516, 1984
28. Bargmann, C.I., Hung, M.-C., and Weinberg, R.A. Cell 45:649-657, 1986
29. Muller, W.J., Sinn, E., Pattengale, P.K., Wallace, R., and Leder, P. Cell 54:105-115, 1988
30. Sinn, E., Muller, W., Pattengale, P., Tepler, I., Wallace, R., and Leder, P. Cell 49:465-475, 1987
31. Andres, A.-C., van der Valk, M.A., Schöenenberger, C.-A., Flückiger, F., LeMeur, M., Gerlinger, P., and Groner, B. Genes Develop. 2:1486-1495, 1988
32. Brinster, R.L., Allen, J.M., Behringer, R.R., Gelinas, R.F., and Palmiter, R.D. Proc. Natl. Acad. Sci. USA 85:836-840, 1988

3

THE CURRENT STATUS OF *int* GENES, PROTO-ONCOGENES, AND RECESSIVE
MUTATIONS IN PRIMARY HUMAN BREAST TUMORS: THEIR POTENTIAL
USEFULNESS IN PROGNOSIS

R. CALLAHAN,[1] I. ALI,[1] K. HACENE,[2] M. BRUNET,[2] R. LIDEREAU[2]

[1]National Cancer Institute, Bethesda, Maryland 20892; [2]Centre René
Huguenin, St. Cloud, France

INTRODUCTION

The diverse biological behavior of breast cancer is thought to
reflect a complex interplay between the physiological status of the
patient and the selection of somatic mutations in mammary epithelium
that either deregulate normal development or provide growth
advantage to tumor cells. One consequence of this biological
diversity has been the difficulty in identifying patients who should
undergo aggressive postsurgical therapy and the nature of the
therapy. Currently, several characteristics of the tumor are used
as indicators of the patient's prognosis. Some of these include
histopathological grade of the tumor, tumor size, and the presence
or absence of estrogen (ER) and progesterone receptors (PR) on the
tumor cells. Presently, the best indicator of patient prognosis is
the extent of tumor involvement in the regional lymph nodes.
However, ≥20% of the lymph node-negative patients will relapse
within 5 yr. Similarly, approximately 50% of the stage II patients
will not respond to postsurgical therapy. This situation highlights
the need for additional independent indicators that can be used to
identify the high-risk patient groups.

During the past few years, we and others have begun to explore
the possibility that specific genetic alterations may be linked to
the more aggressive breast tumors and thus, potentially, to patient
prognosis. In general, these studies have focused on panels of
primary breast tumor DNAs for which information is available on
patient history, tumor characteristics, and postsurgical disease-
free interval of the patient (reviewed in refs. 1 and 2). The types

of mutations frequently found in primary breast tumor DNA fall into
two categories: (a) the quantitative activation of dominant acting
proto-oncogenes and (b) loss of heterozygosity (LOH) at specific
regions of the cellular genome in tumor biopsy material. LOH is
thought to unmask recessive mutations in tumor suppressor genes (3).
Although recombinant clones of only one tumor suppressor gene (Rb-1)
have been obtained (4), it is inferred that there are many of these
genes in the cellular genome. The retinoblastoma gene product
appears to normally suppress cellular proliferation during
development (5). Inactivation of the suppressor gene by point
mutation or deletion allows the cell to escape normal growth
controls.

RESULTS AND DISCUSSION

In our studies, we have focused on a panel of approximately 150
primary breast tumor DNAs for which we have extensive information on
patient history with a median postsurgical follow-up time of 53 mo
(range of 3-127 mo) (6). Presently, we have identified three proto-
oncogenes that are frequently amplified in tumor DNA. In addition,
we have found frequent LOH on chromosomes 3p and 11p in breast tumor
DNA.

Amplification and rearrangement of c-myc.

A study of the c-myc locus in primary breast tumor DNAs from
121 patients revealed two types of genetic alterations (7). In 32%
of the tumors, there was a 2- to 15-fold amplification of the gene.
The amplification was very likely specific for c-myc, because the c-
mos proto-oncogene, also located on chromosome 8, was not amplified.
In five other tumors, a rearrangement of c-myc was detected.
Further analysis of one of these DNAs indicated that the breakpoint
could be near the 3' end of c-myc exon 3. The genetic alteration of
c-myc had a significant correlation ($P < 0.02$) with tumors from
patients ≥51 yr of age. The patients comprising this group either
were postmenopausal, had previously had a hysterectomy (25-30 yr of
age), or were male, suggesting a possible link between their
hormonal milieu and the selection for deregulation of c-myc
expression.

Amplification of c-*myc* and also of other proto-oncogenes is generally associated with enhanced levels of gene expression. Slamon *et al.* (8), using dot blot analysis of RNA from primary breast tumors, noted the frequent expression of c-*myc* RNA. In our study of 14 breast tumor RNA by Northern blot analysis, 10 were found to express high levels of c-*myc* RNA (7). However, only 6 of the 10 tumors contained an amplified c-*myc* gene. It seemed possible that the other four tumors contained mutations outside the restriction fragments examined or contained small undetected mutations that promote c-*myc* RNA expression. One difficulty in evaluating gene expression in total RNA extracted from primary breast tumors is the variable extent of cellular heterogeneity. To circumvent this problem, we have examined c-*myc* expression at the cellular level in frozen sections of breast tumors by using RNA:RNA *in situ* hybridization (9). Positive c-*myc* hybridization signals were associated with carcinoma cells in all cases, including tumors with no apparent alteration of the c-*myc* locus. High levels of c-*myc* expression were observed in four of seven tumors that contained an amplified c-*myc*. Moreover, high levels of c-*myc* RNA were also detected in two of nine cases that had an apparently normal c-*myc* locus but comparatively low cellularity. In addition to carcinoma cells, dense clusters of infiltrating lymphocytes present in three tumors contained c-*myc* RNA. These results, taken together, suggest that (a) the extent and frequency of c-*myc* amplification has probably been underestimated because of heterogeneous cellularity; (b) c-*myc* amplification is related to high level expression, but other unknown factors may also play a role; and (c) c-*myc* RNA in total RNA from biopsy samples may be contributed by infiltrating lymphocytes.

Amplification of the *int*-2 locus.

Recent studies have identified three cellular genetic loci (designated *int*-1, *int*-2, and *int*-3) located on different mouse chromosomes whose expression is activated by mouse mammary tumor virus insertional mutagenesis (10). Activation of *int*-1 is associated with the development of hyperplastic growth of mammary epithelium (11). The *int*-2 gene product is related to basic fibroblast growth factor (FGF) and could therefore promote angiogenesis or delay senescence of mammary epithelium (12). Presently, the organization and nature of the int-3 gene product(s) are being examined.

These considerations have led us to investigate whether the human homologs of the int genes are genetically altered in primary human breast tumors (13). Recombinant clones of human DNA containing int-2-related sequences have recently been obtained and shown to be located on human chromosome 11q13 (14). A survey of 110 primary infiltrating ductal carcinoma DNA showed a 2- to 15-fold amplification of the int-2 locus in 18 tumor DNA. In each of these cases, other loci on chromosome 11p were not amplified, indicating that the amplification was not a result of polyploidy. To characterize the amplification unit containing the int-2 gene, the same panel of breast tumors was screened for possible amplification of other markers mapping between chromosome 11q11 and 11q24 (15). Of eight additional genes analyzed, simultaneous amplification of bcl-1 [11q13, a breakpoint in the t(11;14) translocation in B-cell chronic lymphocytic leukemia] and hst (11q13, another member of the FGF family) was observed in 17 of 18 tumors with an increased copy number of int-2. A single breast tumor showed amplification of int-2 only. Neither bcl-1 nor the hst locus was individually amplified in any of the tumor DNAs examined. These results suggest that amplification of int-2 or a closely linked gene has been selected during tumor development. Examination of patient history, tumor characteristics, and patient prognosis showed that amplification of int-2 had a significant association ($P < 2 \times 10^{-6}$) with the patients who subsequently developed a local recurrence or a distal metastasis.

Currently, there is little available information on the activation of int-2 or hst expression by gene amplification in primary breast tumors. We have used RNA:RNA in situ hybridization to detect int-2 and hst RNA in frozen sections from two primary breast tumors and, in one case, a matching metastatic lymph node (16). In each case, int-2 but not hst RNA was detected. In addition, no int-2 RNA could be detected in normal breast tissue from pregnant women or in breast tumors not containing an amplification of *int*-2. These results were confirmed by Northern blot analysis of RNA from one of the primary breast tumors scoring positive for *int*-2 RNA by *in situ* hybridization. In this case, four species of *int*-2 RNA were detected (4.6, 4.0, 2.6, and 2.0 kb). To further establish the link between *int*-2 gene amplification and expression, additional studies are required.

Amplification of c-*erb*B-2.

The oncogene *neu* was originally identified in chemically induced rat neuroglioblastomas (17). Nucleotide sequence analysis showed it to be related to the c-*erb*B proto-oncogene that encodes the epidermal growth factor receptor (18). The human homolog has been independently identified by several laboratories and designated either HER-2 or c-*erb*B-2 (19-21). The c-*erb*B-2 proto-oncogene is located on chromosome 17q21-22 (22).

We detected a 2- to 40-fold increase in the copy number of the c-*erb*B-2 proto-oncogene in 10% of the panel of primary human breast tumors analyzed (23). The presence of a normal copy number of the gene encoding the tumor antigen p53 (chromosome 17p) provides evidence that the increased copy number of the c-*erb*B-2 gene in certain tumors was due to the amplification of the region containing this proto-oncogene and not to ploidy of chromosome 17. There was no evidence of an association between the amplification of c-*erb*B-2 proto-oncogene and other clinical parameters reflecting the malignancy of the disease, such as the number of involved lymph nodes, age of patients at diagnosis, menopausal status, histopathologic grading of tumors, or hormonal receptor status.

If the amplification of the c-*erb*B-2 proto-oncogene is the hallmark of biologically aggressive breast tumors and confers a selective advantage on the growth and progression of the tumor cells, then subsequent metastases might be expected to also contain a high copy number of this proto-oncogene. Alternatively, amplification of c-*erb*B-2 in the primary tumor but not the metastasis would be consistent with a heterogeneous composition of the primary tumor and the presence of more malignant cells in the metastasis having a normal copy number of the c-*erb*B-2 gene. These contrasting hypotheses were tested by analyzing the c-erbB-2 proto-oncogene in a separate panel of matched sets of DNA from the primary tumors and the corresponding nodal metastases from the same patients (23). A comparable level of c-erbB-2 amplification was observed in the lymph node metastasis of one patient (880M). However, no c-erbB-2 amplification was detected in the lymph node metastasis of another patient, 1043M, suggesting that the increased copy number of the c-erbB-2 proto-oncogene, at least in this patient, may not be a necessary feature of the more malignant tumor cell population. This modality is consistent with our finding that the amplification of c-erbB-2 has not displayed an aggressive biological behavior.

Our observations (23, 24) are in some ways inconsistent with those reported by Slamon et al. (25). First, amplification of c-erbB-2 was detected in 10% of the breast tumors compared with 18 and 40% in two different groups of patients examined by Slamon et al. (25). This difference could in part be due to an underestimation of the copy number of the c-erbB-2 gene because of the presence of contaminating stromal tissue and infiltrating lymphocytes. Conversely, chromosomal duplication rather than gene amplification, at least in some cases, may give rise to an exaggerated frequency of tumors with c-erbB-2 amplification. In our study, we ruled out the latter possibility.

Presently, a simple explanation for these contradictory findings cannot be found. The discrepancies between our results (23, 24) and those of Slamon et al. (25) or among the results of various patient groups studied in the same or different laboratories could reflect differences in genetic background, geographical location, or nutritional and environmental factors (26-31). In this respect, breast cancer patients in the French population seem to have longer disease-free and overall survival periods than the American patients (23). Our results therefore advise caution in the preliminary assignment of c-erbB-2 amplification as an indicator for breast tumor aggressiveness and poor disease prognosis.

Deletion of sequences on chromosomes 3 and 11 in primary breast
tumors.

In a survey of 104 breast cancer patients, deletions of a c-H-
ras-1 allele were detected in 27% of the tumor DNAs of patients
constitutionally heterozygous at this locus (32). To determine the
extent of deletion on chromosome 11 in these tumors, four other
markers [γ globin, parathyroid hormone (PTH), calcitonin, and
catalase] on 11p and the int-2 locus on 11q were examined in matched
sets of lymphocyte and tumor DNA (33). Restriction fragment length
polymorphism analyses using these polymorphic markers demonstrated
that the deletions in breast tumors included, in addition to the c-
H-ras-1 locus, several other loci on chromosome 11. Also, the
deletions were of variable lengths and lacked any apparent common
breakpoint at either end. However, the region of chromosome 11p
that might be critical in these tumors was suggested by the
genotypes of the tumors from two patients that were constitutionally
heterozygous at the c-H-ras-1 locus, the γ locus of the β globin
cluster, and the PTH locus. The tumor DNA from one patient was
reduced to homozygosity at the c-H-ras-1 and γ globin loci but not
at the PTH locus. Conversely, the tumor DNA from the other patient
had lost one PTH allele but maintained heterozygosity at the γ
globin locus. This suggests that a locus located between the β
globin cluster and the PTH locus is important in the development of
breast cancer. Taken together, 20 of 99 tumor DNA examined in our
study (33) exhibited deletions of various markers on chromosome 11p.
These deletions were found to have a significant association with
histopathological grade III ($P < 0.006$) and ER- ($P < 0.02$) and PR-
($P < 0.002$) negative tumors. Other studies have shown that patients
with PR-negative tumors respond poorly to adjuvant endocrine therapy
(34).

In a similar study, we examined four polymorphic markers
(RAF-1, c-erbB-2, c-erbAβ, and DNF 1552) on the short arm and two
polymorphic markers (D3S1 and PCCB) on the long arm of chromosome 3
in 172 breast tumors (35). Twenty-five of the 84 tumors from
constitutionally heterozygous patients were hemizygous at one or
more chromosome 3 loci. Although the deletions were variable in

length, the shortest region of hemizygosity in the tumor DNA was located between the RAF-1 and DNF 1552 loci on the short arm of chromosome 3. This region of chromosome 3 contains at least two members (c-erbA-2 and c-erbAβ) of the steroid/thyroid hormone receptor gene family. This may be particularly pertinent, since LOH on chromosome 3p is associated with ER-negative tumors (χ^2 = 5.44; P < 0.019). In addition, this type of mutation is also associated with histopathological grade III tumors (χ^2 = 18.40; P < 0.0001).

The LOH on chromosomes 3p and 11p is not unique to primary breast tumors. In the case of chromosome 3p, it is also found in lung cancers (36, 37) as well as hereditary and sporadic forms of renal cell carcinomas (38, 39). In addition, chromosome 3p probably contains a locus for the von Hippel-Lindau disease with inherited susceptibility to multiple cancers (40). Similarly, LOH for chromosome 11p is frequently seen in Wilms' tumor (41-45), lung cancer (46), bladder carcinoma (47), and rhabdomyosarcoma (48). The frequency of this type of mutation on chromosomes 3p and 11p suggests the presence of regulatory genes with possible "suppressor" functions. In this regard, various somatic cell hybrid experiments have provided evidence that implicates sequences on the short arm of chromosome 11 in the suppression of tumorigenicity of HeLa cells, a cell line of epithelial origin (49, 50). Since the Wilms' tumor locus (51, 52) appears to be centromeric to the putative breast tumor locus on chromosome 11p, there could be several "suppressor" genes specific for different neoplasias in this region of the genome. Clearly, an expanded study of additional tumors is warranted to focus on the identification and characterization of the affected genes on chromosomes 3p and 11p.

The biological diversity of human breast cancer suggests that multiple mutations are involved in the initiation and progression of the disease. We have observed that 19 of the 25 patients with LOH on chromosome 3 were informative for chromosome 11 markers (35). Consistent with this thesis, 10 of the 19 tumors (53%) also suffered LOH on chromosome 11 in the tumor DNA. In addition, 9 of the 16 tumors (56%) with LOH on chromosome 3p that were tested contained an amplification of c-myc, whereas amplification of c-erbB-2 and int-2 occurred less frequently (10 and 19%, respectively). It seems likely that as our analysis continues, different subgroups of tumors will be identified that can be characterized by the presence of specific sets of mutated genes. Thus, it may be possible to delineate different pathways of mutations that are more closely associated with particular clinical parameters, including patient prognosis, than the individual mutations mentioned above.

Table 1 summarizes the genetic alterations that have been detected in our panel of primary breast tumors and the clinical parameters with which they are associated. In addition, mutations have been identified less frequently at the c-erbA-1 (5%), c-erbB (2%), and c-myb (<1%) loci. No mutations have been detected at the c-K-ras-2, N-ras, N-myc, c-sis, c-mos, ets-1, c-sea, p53, int-1, met-H, c-erbB-1, and somatostatin loci.

Table 1. Summary of mutations in primary breast tumors.

Gene(s) (chromosome)	Type of mutation	Frequency (%)	Associated clinical parameters
c-myc (8q)	Amplification (or rearrangement)	32 (4)	Patients ≥51 yr of age
c-erbB-2 (17q)	Amplification	10	None
int-2 (11q)	Amplification	16	Local recurrence or distal metastasis
(11p)	Deletion	20	ER/PR-negative tumors, histopath. grade III tumors
(3p)	Deletion	30	ER-negative tumors, histopath. grade III tumors

Association between prognosis and breast tumor mutations in different subgroups of patients.

Recently, we have begun to re-examine our data to determine whether, in certain subgroups of patients defined by clinical parameters, specific mutations distinguish patients with a poor prognosis (53). To accomplish this, we have focused on 129 of the previously described tumors for which complete information was available on the patient and the tumor. In addition, we eliminated from consideration patients with (a) two different kinds of simultaneously occurring tumors or two contralateral breast tumors, (b) male breast tumors, and (c) local recurrent tumors. In the present study, only metastasis was considered in determining associations between a mutation and prognosis. As in our previous analysis, the median follow-up time on the patients was 53 mo (range of 3-127 mo). Significant prognostic relationships were identified by univariate log rank analysis (54). The highlights of this analysis showed that tumors having the following characteristics and mutations were associated with poor postsurgical prognosis: (a) premenopausal patients with either an amplification of c-*myc* ($P < 0.0097$) or *int*-2 ($P < 0.0093$), (b) postmenopausal patients with LOH at c-*erb*A-2 (chromosome 3p) ($P < 0.026$), (c) lymph node-positive patients with an amplification of *int*-2 ($P < 0.0016$) or LOH at c-*erb*A-2 ($P < 0.0066$), and (d) ER- and PR-negative tumors having an amplification of *int*-2 ($P < 0.0127$ and $P < 0.001$, respectively) or LOH at c-*erb*A-2 ($P < 0.0031$ and $P < 0.0088$, respectively). Amplification of c-*erb*B-2 or LOH at c-H-*ras*-1 (chromosome 11p) was not associated with patient prognosis in the categories studied.

Multivariate Cox regression analysis showed that in the tumors tested for *int*-2 gene amplification, PR-negative tumors ($P < 0.0019$) and tumors containing an amplified *int*-2 gene ($P < 0.018$) represented independent prognosis parameters (55). Moreover, it was possible to develop four risk classes using these two parameters. As shown in Table 2, the risk for patients whose tumor is PR negative is 5-fold higher if *int*-2 is amplified. Similarly, the risk is 10-fold higher than in patients with PR-positive tumors irrespective of *int*-2 gene amplification.

Our results and those of other laboratories (reviewed in refs. 1 and 2) point to the hypothesis that specific mutations may be useful prognostic indicators of the postsurgical course of the disease in breast cancer patients. However, there are significant

Table 2. Risk factors for patients tested for *int-2* gene
amplification.

Class	Number of patients	Number of relapses (%)	Risk factors	*P* values
1 PR$^+$ Amp$^+$	6	1 (17)	1.00	
2 PR$^+$ Amp$^-$	44	8 (18)	1.10	
3 PR$^-$ Amp$^-$	33	12 (36)	2.56	
4 PR$^-$ Amp$^+$	7	6 (86)	11.80	0.0000026

variations in the results of different studies. Some factors that
may contribute to the conflicting reports on associations between
specific genetic alterations and patient prognosis are that (a) some
studies had only a limited period of postsurgical follow up while in
others the follow up spanned several months to 10 yr; (b) in some
studies, inappropriate statistical methodology was used in the
treatment of the data; (c) differences in the sensitivity and
quantifiable aspects of the techniques used to measure the levels of
expression or copy number of the gene in biopsy material provided
other confounding factors in comparing the statistical treatment of
the respective data; and (d) associations between particular
mutations and patient relapse or survival were determined without
considering the postsurgical treatment received by the patient.
These factors clearly demonstrate the need for confirmation of
putative prognostic genetic alterations on much larger panels of
tumors. The major difficulty in undertaking retrospective studies
of primary breast tumor DNA is the scarcity of frozen tumor and
normal biopsy material from surgeries performed 5-10 yr ago for
which follow-up data on the patients' disease statuses are
available. Similarly, a serious attempt to study less frequently
occurring histopathological types of breast carcinomas has been
significantly impeded. The recent development of techniques that
lead to the recovery of DNA from formalin-fixed tissue specimens
embedded in paraffin could provide an additional resource given the
vast archives of tumor specimens in pathology departments throughout
the world (56, 57). Similarly, the polymerase chain reaction has

been successfully used to amplify cellular DNA in thin sections of
formalin-fixed paraffin-embedded tissue specimens that are up to 40
yr old (58, 59). Taken together, these new approaches may provide a
clearer picture of the usefulness of genetic alterations as
prognostic indicators.

REFERENCES

1. Callahan, R. Breast Cancer Res. Treat., in press, 1989.
2. Ali, I.U. and Callahan, R. In: Molecular Genetics and the
   Diagnosis of Cancer (Ed. J. Cossman), Elsevier, New York, 1989,
   in press.
3. Knudson, A.G. Proc. Natl. Acad. Sci. USA 68: 820-823, 1971.
4. Friend, S.H., Horowitz, J.M., Gerber, M.R., Wang, X.-F.,
   Bogenmann, E., Li, F.P. and Weinberg, R.A. Proc. Natl. Acad.
   Sci. USA 84: 9059-9063, 1987.
5. Huang, H.-J.S., Yee, J.-K., Shew, J.-Y., Chen, P.-L.,
   Bookstein, R., Friedmann, T., Lee, E.Y.-H.P. and Lee, W.-H.
   Science 242: 1563-1566, 1988.
6. Lidereau, R., Escot, C., Theillet, C., Champeme, M.H., Brunet,
   M., Gest, J. and Callahan, R. J. Natl. Cancer Inst. 77: 697-
   701, 1986.
7. Escot, C., Theillet, C., Lidereau, R., Spyratos, F., Champeme,
   M.H., Gest, J. and Callahan, R. Proc. Natl. Acad. Sci. USA 83:
   4834-4838, 1986.
8. Slamon, D.J., de Kernion, J.B., Verma, I.M. and Cline, M.J.
   Science 224: 256-262, 1984.
9. Mariani-Costantini, R., Escot, C., Theillet, C., Gentile, A.,
   Merlo, G., Lidereau, R. and Callahan, R. Cancer Res. 48: 199-
   205, 1988.
10. Callahan, R. In: The Mammary Gland: Development, Regulation
    and Function (Eds. M.C. Neville and C. Daniel), Plenum, New
    York, 1987, pp. 323-351.
11. Tsukamoto, A.S., Grosschedl, R., Guzman, R.C., Parslow, T. and
    Varmus, H.E. Cell 55: 619-625, 1988.
12. Dickson, C. and Peters, G. Nature 326: 833, 1987.
13. Lidereau, R., Callahan, R., Dickson, C., Peters, G., Escot, C.
    and Ali, I.U. Oncogene Res. 2: 285-291, 1988.
14. Casey, G., Smith, R., McGillivray, D., Peters, G. and Dickson,
    C. Mol. Cell. Biol. 6: 502-510, 1986.
15. Ali, I.U., Merlo, G., Lidereau, R. and Callahan, R. Oncogene
    4: 89-92, 1989.
16. Liscia, D.S., Merlo, G.R., Garrett, C., Mariani-Costantini, R.,
    French, P. and Callahan, R. Manuscript in preparation.
17. Shih, C., Padney, L., Murray, M. and Weinberg, R.A. Nature
    290: 261-264, 1981.
18. Bargmann, C.I., Hung, M.C. and Weinberg, R.A. Cell 45: 649-
    657, 1986.
19. King, C.R., Kraus, M.H. and Aaronson, S.A. Science 229: 974-
    976, 1985.
20. Semba, K., Kamata, N., Toyoshima, F. and Yamamoto, T. Proc.
    Natl. Acad. Sci. USA 82: 6497-6501, 1985.

21. Schechter, A.L., Stern, D.F., Valdyanathan, L., Decker, S.J., Drebin, J.A., Greene, M.E. and Weinberg, R.A. Nature 312: 513-516, 1984.
22. Fukushige, S.I., Mastsubara, K.I., Yoshida, M., Sasaki, M., Suzuki, T., Semba, K., Toyoshima, K. and Yamamoto, T. Mol. Cell. Biol. 6: 955-958, 1986.
23. Ali, I.U., Campbell, G., Lidereau, R. and Callahan, R. Oncogene Res. 3: 139-146, 1988.
24. Ali, I.U., Campbell, G., Lidereau, R. and Callahan, R. Science 240: 1795-1796.
25. Slamon, D.J., Clark, G.M., Wong, S.G., Levin, W.S., Ullrich, A. and McGuire, W.L. Science 235: 177-182, 1987.
26. Varley, J.M., Swallow, J.E., Brammar, W.J., Whittaker, J.L. and Walker, R.A. Oncogene 1: 423-430, 1987.
27. Guerin, M., Barrois, M., Terrier, M.J., Spielmann, M. and Riou, G. Oncogene Res. 3: 21-31, 1988.
28. van de Vijver, M., van de Bersselaur, R., Devilee, P., Cornelisse, C., Peterse, J. and Nusse, R. Mol. Cell. Biol. 7: 2019-2023, 1987.
29. Zhou, D., Battifora, H., Yokota, J., Yamamoto, T. and Cline, M.J. Cancer Res. 47: 6123-6125, 1987.
30. Venter, D.J., Tuzi, N.L., Kumar, S. and Gullick, W.J. Lancet ii: 69-72, 1987.
31. Berger, M.S., Locher, G.W., Sauer, S., Gullick, W.J., Waterfield, M.D., Groner, B. and Hynes, N.E. Cancer Res. 48: 1238-1243, 1988.
32. Theillet, C., Lidereau, R., Escot, C., Hutzell, P., Brunet, M., Gest, J., Schlom, J. and Callahan, R. Cancer Res. 46: 4776-4781, 1986.
33. Ali, I.U., Lidereau, R., Theillet, C. and Callahan, R. Science 238: 185-188, 1987.
34. McGuire, W.L. Cancer Surv. 5: 527-531, 1986.
35. Ali, I.U., Lidereau, R. and Callahan, R. Manuscript in preparation.
36. Yokota, J., Wada, M., Shimosato, Y., Terada, M. and Sugimura, T. Proc. Natl. Acad. Sci. USA 84: 9252-9256, 1987.
37. Naylor, S.L., Johnson, B.E., Minna, J.D. and Sakaguchi, A.Y. Nature 329: 451-454, 1987.
38. Kovacs, G., Erlandsson, R., Boldog, F., Ingvarsson, F., Müller-Brechlin, R., Klein, G. and Sümegi, J. Proc. Natl. Acad. Sci. USA 85: 1571-1575, 1988.
39. Zbar, B., Branch, H., Talmadge, C. and Linehan, M. Nature 327: 721-724, 1987.
40. Seizinger, B.R., Rouleau, G.A., Ozelius, L.J., et al. Nature 332: 268-269, 1988.
41. Riccardi, V. M., Sujansky, E., Smith, A.C. and Franke, U. Pediatrics 61: 604-610, 1978.
42. Koufos, A., Hansen, M.F., Lampkin, B.C., Workman, M.L., Copeland, N.G., Jenkins, N.A. and Cavence, W.K. Nature 309: 170-172, 1984.
43. Orkin, S.H., Goldman, D.S. and Sallan, S.E. Nature 309: 172-174, 1984.
44. Reeve, A.E., Harsiaux, P.J., Gardner, R.J.M., Chewings, W.E., Grindley, R.M. and Millow, L.J. Nature 309: 174-176, 1984.

45. Fearon, E.R., Vogelstein, B. and Feinberg, A.P. Nature 309: 176-178, 1984.
46. Shiraishi, M., Morinaga, S., Noguchi, M., Shimosato, Y. and Sekiya, T. Jpn. J. Cancer Res. 78: 1302-1308, 1987.
47. Fearon, E.R., Feinberg, A.P., Hamilton, S.H. and Vogelstein, B. Nature 318: 377-380, 1985.
48. Scrable, H.J., Witte, D.P., Lampkin, B.C. and Cavenee, W.K. Nature 329: 645-647, 1987.
49. Stanbridge, E.J., Flandermeyer, R.R., Daniels, D.W. and Nelson-Rees, W.A. Somatic Cell Genet. 7: 699-709, 1981.
50. Kaebling, M. and Klinger, H.P. Cytogenet. Cell Genet. 41: 65-70, 1985.
51. Raizis, A.M., Becroft, D.M., Shaw, R.L. and Reeve, A.E. Hum. Genet. 70: 344-346, 1985.
52. Glaser, T., Lewis, W.H., Bruns, G.A.P., Watkins, P.C., Rogler, C.E., Shows, T.B., Power, V.E., Willard, H.F., Goguen, J.M., Simola, O.J. and Housman, D.E. Nature 321: 882-887, 1986.
53. Lidereau, R., Champeme, M.H., Ali, I., Brunet, M., Callahan, R., Escot, C., Theillet, C. and Hacene, K. Manuscript in preparation.
54. Peto, R., Pike, M.C., Armitage, P., et al. Br. J. Cancer 35: 1-39, 1977.
55. Lidereau, R., Champeme, M.H., Ali, I., Callahan, R., Escot, C., Hacene, K., Theillet, C. and Brunet, M. Manuscript in preparation.
56. Goelz, S.E., Hamilton, S.R. and Vogelstein, B. Biochem. Biophys. Res. Commun. 130: 118-126, 1985.
57. Dubeau, L., Chandler, L.A., Gralow, J.R., Nichols, P.W. and Jones, P.A. Cancer Res. 46: 2964-2969, 1986.
58. Saiki, R.K., Gelfand, D.H., Stoffel, S., Scharf, S.J., Higuchi, R., Horn, G.T., Mullis, E.B. and Erlich, H.A. Science 239: 487-491, 1988.
59. Shibata, D., Martin, W.J. and Arnheim, N. Cancer Res. 48: 4564-4566, 1988.

4

ISOLATION AND CHARACTERIZATION OF FULL LENGTH cDNA CODING FOR THE H23
BREAST TUMOR ASSOCIATED ANTIGEN

D.H. Wreschner, I.Tsarfaty, M. Hareuveni, J. Zaretsky, N. Smorodinsky,
M. Weiss, J. Horev, P. Kotkes, S. Zrihan, J.M. Jeltsch[*], S. Green[*],
R. Lathe[*] and I. Keydar

Department of Microbiology, Tel Aviv University, Ramat Aviv, Israel
and [*]LGME-CNRS and U184-Inserm, Strasbourg, France

ABSTRACT

A monoclonal antibody, H23, that specifically recognizes a breast
tumor associated antigen(H23 Ag) was used to isolate a cDNA insert
that codes for the antigenic epitope. Nucleotide sequencing of this
cDNA as well as a longer 850 bp cDNA insert showed that they are composed of highly conserved 60 bp G + C rich tandem repeating units.
Full length cDNAs that code for the H23 Ag were isolated by reprobing
the cDNA library with unique sequence genomic fragments. The longest
open reading frame (ORF) defines a serine rich protein that can be
conveniently divided into 3 regions. The first region (127 a.a.)
contains an initiating methionine and highly hydrophobic signal peptide. This is followed by a variable number (20-80x)of a 20 amino
acid repeat that is rich in proline, alanine, threonine, serine and
glycine. The last region, comprising 160 a.a. is situated on the
COOH side of the repeat array and contains 4 potential N-linked
glycosylation sites. The availability of full length cDNA now permits the design of experiments intended to clarify the role of H23 Ag
in the development of breast cancer.

INTRODUCTION

The identification and characterization of antigens that are
overexpressed in human breast cancer may lead to new therapeutic,
prognostic and diagnostic avenues. Many groups have directed much
effort towards this goal and the literature is replete with reports
describing the production of a number of different monoclonal antibodies (MoAbs) that bind to an antigen of epithelial cell origin that
is apparently overexpressed in breast cancer cells (1-10). A variety

of immunogens including cell membranes of metastatic breast tumor cells, human milk fat globules, deglycosylated mucin and particulate proteins released by breast tumor cells have been used to elicit these MoAbs. Whereas some of these antibodies recognize antigens both on normal and tumor epithelial tissue, other MoAbs demonstrate a remarkable specificity for cells of breast cancer origin (1, 11).

The general picture that emerges is that many, if not all, of these MoAbs are recognizing highly similar antigens that probably have quantitative and qualitative differences depending on whether they are expressed in normal or tumor tissues.

We have recently reported the production of a MoAb, H23, that specifically stains the cytoplasm of 92% of breast cancer tissue sections as detected by immunohistochemical staining (1). In contrast, normal or benign breast tissue did not show any intracellular staining and, if present, the location of antigen was apical or/and intraductal.

Furthermore, the antigen (designated H23 Ag) could be detected in body fluids, and the serum antigen levels in breast cancer patients correlates with the prognosis of the disease (12).

In order to learn more about its increased expression and possible role in breast cancer, we embarked on a molecular analysis of the H23 antigen. We present here the isolation and characterization of full length cDNA that codes for this potentially useful breast cancer marker.

MATERIALS AND METHODS

Isolation of Monoclonal Antibodies.

Monoclonal antibodies were generated against particulate proteins released into the culture medium by T47D breast cancer cells using established techniques (1). Supernatants of the hybridomas obtained were screened by immunohistochemical staining of breast tissue paraffin sections and one MoAb, specifically stained the cytoplasm of breast tumor tissue. This MoAb, designated H23, was used for further study.

Screening of gtll cDNA library.

A gtll cDNA expression library prepared with mRNA isolated from T47D breast cancer cells (13) was screened with H23 MoAbs and positive plaques purified to homogeneity. The cDNA inserts were isolated and subcloned into pβR322 and M13 sequencing vectors.

Isolation of genomic fragment coding for the H23 Antigen.

The isolated cDNA insert obtained above was used to screen a genomic library prepared in λwes with EcoRl restricted DNA that had been isolated from MCF7 breast cancer. Positive recombinants were purified to homogeneity and a 7.5 kb genomic fragment thus isolated was subcloned into puN121.

Isolation of full length cDNAs.

Selected genomic fragments that did not contain the 60bp repeat unit (see Results section) but nonetheless hybridized with identical mRNA species as the original 60bp repeat cDNA inserts (see Results) were used to reprobe the gtll T47D cDNA library. The cDNA inserts obtained were subcloned into pGEM1 and M-13 sequencing vectors.

Nucleotide sequencing.

Restriction fragments derived from cloned cDNAs were subcloned into M13 vectors and the nucleotide sequence determined on the ssDNA template by the dideoxy method (14).

RESULTS

Isolation of cDNA inserts containing 60bp repeat units. Screening of the gtll T47D cDNA expression library with the H23 MoAbs resulted in positive recombinants that appeared at a frequency of approximately 1 in 2-4,000 phages in the amplified library. The longest cDNA, designated 3b, was 225 bp in length and this insert was used to rescreen the cDNA library. A longer 850 bp cDNA was isolated and the nucleotide sequence determined for both the original 3b and the longer 850 bp cDNA insert. The sequence indicated that both these cDNAs were completely composed of almost perfect tandem 60 bp repeat units. A comparison of the individual repeats with the consensus 60 bp repeat motif showed very high conservation of the G + C rich nucleotide sequence with a maximum of 4 nucleotide substitutions in any one repeat unit. The locations of these nucleotide substitutions did not occur randomly but were rather clustered at certain positions within the consensus repeat motifs (Fig. 1).

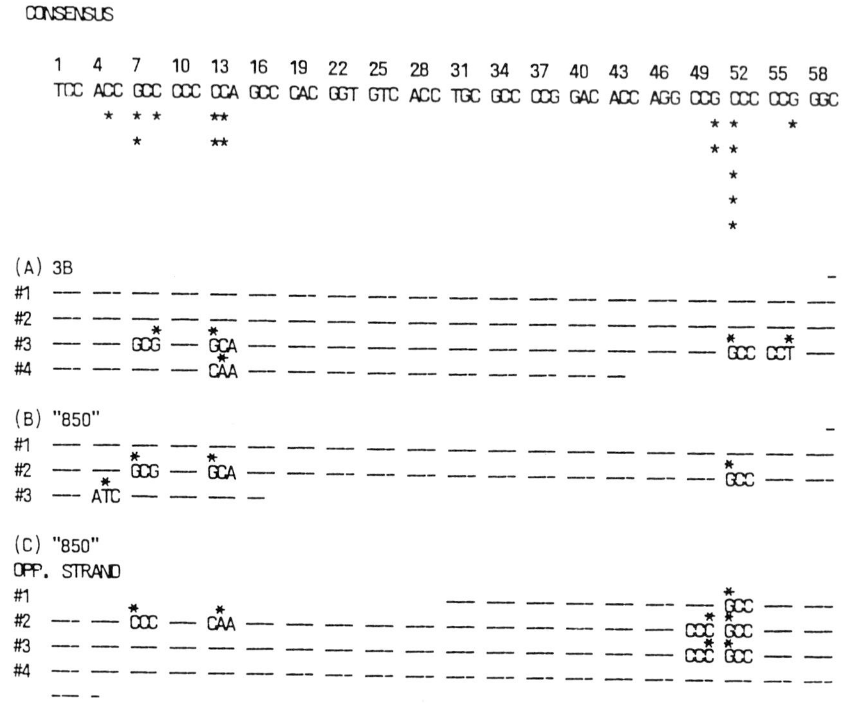

CONSENSUS

Figure 1: <u>Nucleotide sequence of cDNAs that code for the epitope recognized by H23 MoAbs and contain tandem repeat 60 bp units.</u>

The λgt11 cDNA expression library was screened with H23 MoAbs as described in Methods and the cDNA insert ("3b") obtained from a positive purified recombinant phage was subcloned in M13 vectors in both orientations and sequenced (Fig. 1A). The 3b cDNA insert was purified, nick translated and used to reprobe the library under stringent hybridization conditions as described in Methods. The longest cDNA insert (850 bp) thus obtained was subcloned in M13 and both strands were partially sequenced (Figs. 1B and C). Only the "C" rich strand is presented. The consensus sequence of the 60bp repeat unit is shown at the top of the figure. Nucleotides in the repeat units identical to this sequence are indicated with dashes whilst substitutions are shown by an asterisk.

Coding strand of the repeat motif and its overexpression in breast cancer tissue.

In order to determine the coding strand of the 60 bp repeat unit a synthetic oligonucleotide and its complementary oligonucleotide corresponding to nucleotides 15 to 43 in the consensus sequence were synthesized and used to probe Northern blots containing RNA isolated from tumor breast tissue and adjacent "normal" breast tissue. Whereas no hybridization was observed with "C" rich oligonucleotide, the "G" rich complementary oligonucleotide demonstrated an identical pattern of hybridization to that seen with the complete 3b cDNA insert, thus indicating that the coding strand of the repeat motif is the "C" rich strand (Fig. 2).

The RNA isolated from malignant breast tissues contained in the one case a 3.6 kb hybridizing mRNA species whilst the second sample showed a 6.5 kb hybridizing band. The corresponding adjacent "normal" breast tissues had much reduced levels of hybridizing mRNAs (Fig. 2).

An extensive RNA analysis from additional breast tissues confirmed that 3b hybridizing mRNA species were overexpressed in malignant breast tissue as compared to the corresponding adjacent "normal" breast tissue.

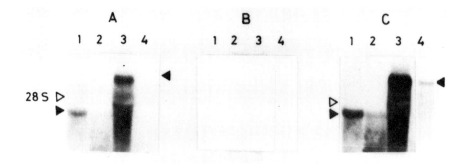

Figure 2.   Northern blot analysis of human breast tumor RNA
samples with 3b cDNA probe and synthetic complementary oligonucleo-
tides derived from the repeating unit.

RNA was extracted from human breast tumor tissue or adjacent
"normal" breast tissue (lanes 1,3 or 2,4 respectively) from 2 separate individuals (lanes 1,2 and 3.4) and analyzed by glyoxal agarose
gel electrophoresis followed by Northern blotting to Nylon membranes
and hybridization with the 3b cDNA probe (A), with the "C" rich
oligonucleotide 5' AGCCCACGGTGTCACCTCGGCCCCGGACA3' identical to
nucleotides 15 to 43 of the concensus sequence presented in Fig. 1A
and the complementary "G" rich oligo-nucleotide 5' TGTCCGGGGCCGAGGTG
ACACCGTGGGCT3' (C). The probe used in (A) was radioactively label-

led by nick translation whilst those used in (B) and (C) were end labelled by polynucleotide kinase and ATP as described in Methods. The blots were stringently washed and autoradiographed at -70 degrees C. The full arrow to the left of the figure indicates the 3.6 kb hybridizing mRNA species whilst that on the right points to the 6.0Kb mRNA species detected in the other sample. The open arrow indicates the position of 28S rRNA.

Multiple mRNA species expressed correspond to the different poly-morphic allelic forms of a VNTR gene.

The remarkable structure of tandem 60 bp repeat units observed in the isolated cDNAs suggested expression of a gene that contains a variable number of tandem repeats (VNTRs). Such genes are known to be highly polymorphic (15,16) and Southern blot analyses performed on DNA extracted from primary human tumors indeed demonstrated marked polymorphism when probed with 3b cDNA (Fig. 3A). Most samples tested were heterozygous and many differently sized alleles could be observed. The heterogeneity in allelic sizes could be directly attributed to differences in the number of 60 bp repeat units present within the repeat array of each allele, as reprobing the same Southern blot with a non-repeat genomic fragment derived from the isolated gene hybridized with a unique identical band in all samples analyzed (Fig. 3B).

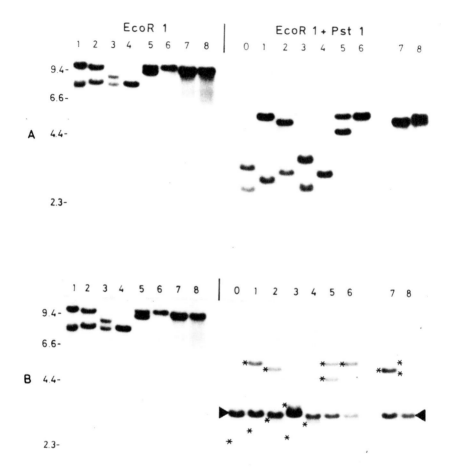

Figure 3. <u>Hybridization of Southern blots with the repeating unit</u>
<u>unit demonstrates a highly polymorphic gene.</u>

High molecular weight genomic DNA was extracted from human
epithelial tumors, restricted with EcoRI alone or doubly digested
with EcoRI and Pst1 and 10 µg was electrophoresed on agarose gels,
Southern blotted and probed with radioactively labelled 850 bp cDNA
(A) and following this hybridization, the blot was rehybridized with
a 1Kb non-repeat fragment of the gene (see Text). The blots were
stringently washed and autoradiographed at -70 degrees C. The bands
labelled in "B" with the asterisk are the remaining signals of those

seen in the previous hybridization with the repeat unit, whilst the specifically labelled band is shown by the full arrows (B, EcoRI + Psti). The numbers to the left of the figure indicate markers in Kilobase pairs.

Probing of Northern blots, containing RNA isolated from the same samples described above, with the 3b cDNA probe demonstrated marked heterogeneity in the hybridizing mRNA species. A complete concordance between the relative mRNA sizes and the corresponding allelic forms in any individual sample, was observed (Fig. 4).

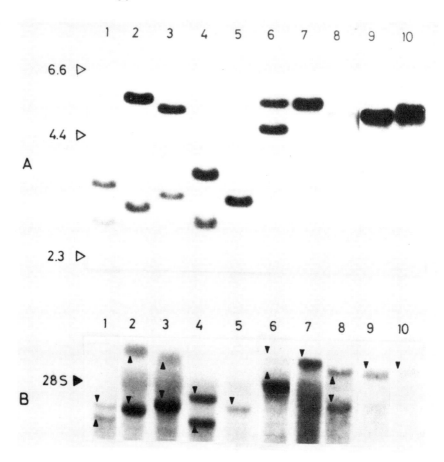

Figure 4. Correlation of Southern and Northern blots containing DNA and RNA isolated from the same human tissue sample following hybridization with the repeating unit.

DNA (A) or total RNA (B) was isolated from human epithelial

tissues. The DNA after double digestion with EcoRI and Pst1 or total
RNA samples were electrophoresed on agarose gels and Southern (A) or
Northern (B) blotted followed by hybridization with radioactively
labelled 3b cDNA probe. The blots were stringently washed and autoradiographed at −70 degrees C. All samples in A were run simultaneously on the same gel but lane 8 was exposed for a longer time as
less DNA was available for analysis. On the Northern blot samples
2 to 7 were run simultaneously on the same gel but lane 6 was exposed for a longer time as there was significantly less mRNA expression in this sample. Samples 1 and samples 8 to 10 were run on
2 separate gels. The positions of the hybridizing mRNA species are
indicated in B by the upward or downward facing full arrows. Note
that in lanes 2 to 7 (and especially in lane 6) nonspecific hybridization with 28S rRNA has occurred.

The patterns of hybridization observed in the Northern and
Southern blots indicated (a) that the gene coding for the H23 antigen
contains a variable number of tandem repeats and can thus be classified as a VNTR gene and (b) that the alleles of the VNTR gene trans-
cribe heterogenously sized mRNAs whose size heterogeneity is a consequence of a variation in the number of tandem repeats.

Nucleotide sequence of full length cDNA.

The above results suggested that 5' and 3' to the 60 bp repeat
array the mRNA coding for the H23 antigen probably contains unique
nucleotide sequences. In order to learn more about the role that
this antigen plays in breast cancer, it was imperative to define
these sequences.

The initial strategy used to obtain cDNA clones that span the
entire mRNA molecule involved reprobing the gt11 cDNA library with
the 60 bp repeat unit. Although a large number (approximately 300)
of positive recombinant phages were identified, nucleotide
sequence analysis of the cDNA inserts from a selected number showed
that they were composed of different multiples of the 60 bp unit.
It was thus apparent that cDNA clones representing unique sequences
of the H23 Ag mRNA appeared only at low frequencies. To resolve
this problem, the cDNA library was reprobed with genomic fragments
located 5' and 3' to the tandem array that although representing

unique genomic sequences nonetheless hybridized with mRNA species identical to those detected with the 60 bp repeat cDNA probe. This approach resulted in the isolation of cDNA inserts that were situated 5' and 3' to the repeat array (Fig. 5, Full Length cDNA).

Figure 5.   Sequence of Full Length cDNA Coding for H23 Ag.
            (See following page)

     cDNA inserts corresponding to regions 5' and 3' of the tandem repeat array were isolated by probing the T47D cDNA library with unique genomic fragments (see Text). These inserts were subcloned into M13 vectors and sequenced by the dideoxy method (14). Synthetic Eco R1 sites used in the production of the cDNAs are located at the 5' and 3' termini. The region corresponding to the putative signal peptide is indicated and boxed in as are the 3 representative 20 amino acid repeat units bounded by Sma 1 sites. The actual repeat array can span from 20 to 80 repeat units. Only one other Sma 1 site appears at nucleotide #1907 (not indicated). Putative N-linked glycosylation sites are shown by *. The nucleotide and amino acid residue numbering appear to the left and right of the figure, respectively.

```
            EcoR1                                   "KOZAK"  Met

  1  GAATTCCCTGGCTGCTTGAATCTGTTCTGCCCCCTCCCCACCCATTTCACCACCACCATG
                                                            ─────── M    1
                                                                     ─

                             SIGNAL PEPTIDE
 61  ACACCGGGCACCCAGTCTCCTTTCTTCCTGCTGCTGCTCCTCACAGTGCTTACAGTTGTT
      T  P  G  T  Q  S  P │ F  F  L  L  L  L  L  T  V  L  T  V  V │  21

121  ACAGGTTCTGGTCATGCAAGCTCTACCCCAGGTGGAGAAAAGGAGACTTCGGCTACCCAG
      T  G  S  G  H  A  S  S  T  P  G  G  E  K  E  T  S  A  T  Q    41
181  AGAAGTTCAGTGCCCAGCTCTACTGAGAAGAATGCTGTGAGTATGACCAGCAGCGTACTC
      R  S  S  V  P  S  S  T  E  K  N  A  V  S  M  T  S  S  V  L    61
241  TCCAGCCACAGCCCCGGTTCAGGCTCCTCCACCACTCAGGGACAGGATGTCACTCTGGCC
      S  S  H  S  P  G  S  G  S  S  T  T  Q  G  Q  D  V  T  L  A    81
301  CCGGCCACGGAACCAGCTTCAGGTTCAGCTGCCACCTGGGGACAGGATGTCACTTCGGTC
      P  A  T  E  P  A  S  G  S  A  A  T  W  G  Q  D  V  T  S  V   101
361  CCAGTCACCAGGCCAGCCCTGGGCTCCACCACCCCGCCAGCCCACGATGTCACCTCAGCC
      P  V  T  R  P  A  L  G  S  T  T  P  P  A  H  D  V  T  S  A   121
                         Sma1           REPEAT UNIT
421  CCGGACAACAAGCCAGCCCCGGGCTCCACCGCCCCCCCAGCCCACGGTGTCACCTCGGCC

      P  D  N  K  P  A │ P  G  S  T  A  P  P  A  H  G  V  T  S  A   141
                 Sma1
481  CCGGACACCAGGCCGCCCCCGGGCTCCACCGCCCCCCCAGCCCACGGTGTCACCTCGGCC

      P  D  T  R  P  P │ P  G  S  T  A  P  P  A  H  G  V  T  S  A   161
                   Sma1
541  CCGGACACCAGGCCGCCCCCGGGCTCCACCGCGCCCGCAGCCCACGGTGTCACCTCGGCC

      P  D  T  R  P  P │ P  G  S  T  A  P  A  A  H  G  V  T  S  A   181
                   Sma1
601  CCGGACACCAGGCCGGCCCCGGGCTCCACCGCCCCCCCAGCCCATGGTGTCACCTCGGCC

      P  D  T  R  P  A │ P  G  S  T  A  P  P  A  H  G  V  T  S  A   201
661  CCGGACAACAGGCCCGCCTTGGGCTCCACCGCCCCTCCAGTCCACAATGTCACCTCGGCC
      P  D  N  R  P  A  L  G  S  T  A  P  P  V  H  N* V  T  S  A   221
721  TCAGGCTCTGCATCAGGCTCAGCTTCTACTCTGGTGCACAACGGCACCTCTGCCCAGGGCT
      S  G  S  A  S  G  S  A  S  T  L  V  H  N* G  T  S  A  R  A   241
781  ACCACAACCCCAGCCAGCAAGAGCACTCCATTCTCAATTCCCAGCCACCACTCTGATACT
      T  T  T  P  A  S  K  S  T  P  F  S  I  P  S  H  H  S  D  T   261
841  CCTACCACCCTTGCCAGCCATAGCACCAAGACTGATGCCAGTAGCACTCACCATAGCACG
      P  T  T  L  A  S  H  S  T  K  T  D  A  S  S  T  H  H  S  T   281
901  GTACCTCCTCTCACCTCCTCCAATCACAGCACTTCTCCCCAGTTGTCTACTGGGGTCTCT
      V  P  P  L  T  S  S  N* H  S  T  S  P  Q  L  S  T  G  V  S   301
961  TTCTTTTTCCTGTCTTTTCACATTTCAAACCTCCAGTTTAATTCCTCTCTGGAAGATCCC
      F  F  F  L  S  F  H  I  S  N  L  Q  F  N* S  S  L  E  D  P   321
1021 AGCACCGACTACTACCAAGAGCTGCAGAGAGACATTTCTGAAATGGTGAGTATCGGCCTT
      S  T  D  Y  Y  Q  E  L  Q  R  D  I  S  E  M  V  S  I  G  L   341
1081 TCCTTCCCCATGCTCCCCTGAAGCAGCCATCAGAACTGTCCACACCCTTTGCATCAAGCC
      S  F  P  M  L  P End                                         347
1141 TGAGTCCTTTCCCTCTCACCCCAGTTTTTGCAGATTTATAAACAAGGGGGTTTTCTGGGC
1201 CTCTCCAATATTAAGTTCAGGTACAGTTCTGGGTGTGGACCCAGTGTGGTGGTTGGAGGG
1261 TTGGGTGGTGGTCATGACCGTAGGAGGGACTGGTCGCACTTAAGGTTGGGGGAAGAGTCG
1321 TGAGCCAGAGCTGGGACCCGTGGCTGAAGTGCCCATTTCCCTGTGACCAGGCCAGGATCT
1381 GTGGTGGTACAATTGACTCTGGCCTTCCGAGAAGGTACCATCAATGTCCACGACGTGGAG
1441 ACACAGTTCAATCAGTATAAAACGGAAGCAGCCTCTCGATATAACCTGACGATCTCAAGA
1501 CGTCAGCGGTGAGGCTACTTCCCTGGCTGCAGCCCAGCACCATGCCGGGGCCCTCTCCTT
1561 CCAGTGCCTGGGTCCCCGCTCTTTCCTTAGTGCTGGCAGCGGGAGGGGGCGCCTCCTCTGG
1621 GAGACTGCCCTGACCACTGCTTTTCCTTTTAGTGAGTGATGTGCCATTTCCTTTCTCTGC
1681 CCAGTCTGGGGCTGGGGTGCCAGGCTGGGGCATCGCGCTGCTGGTGCTGGTCTGTGTTCT
1741 GGTTGCGCTGGCCATTGTCTATCTCATTGCCTTGGTGAGTGCAGTCCCTGGCCCTGATCA
1801 GAGCCCCCCCGGTAGAAGGCACTCCATGGCCTGCCATAACCTCCTATCTCCCCAGGCTGTC
1861 TGTCAGTGCCGCCGAAAGAACTACGGGCAGCTGGACATCTTTCCAGCCCGGGATACCTAC
1921 CATCCTATGAGCGAGTACCCCACCTACCACACCCATGGCGCTATGTGCCCCCCTAGCAGTA
1981 CCGATCGTAGCCCCTATGAGAAGGTGAGATTGGCCCCACAGGCCAGGGGAAGCAGAGGGT
2041 TTGGCTGGGCAAGGATTCTGAAGGGGGTACTTGGAAAACCCAAAGAGCTTGGAAGAGGTG
2101 AGAAGTGGCGTGAAGTGAGCAGGGGAGGGCCTGGAAAGGATGAGGGGCAGAGGTCAGAGG
2161 AGTTTTGGGGGACAGGCCTGGGAGGAGGACTATGGAAGAAAGGGGCCCTCAAAAGGGAGTG
2221 GCCCCACTGCCAGAATTC
```

The longest cDNA insert 5' to the repeat array pse 5, is 520 bp long (including the 5' and 3' synthetic Eco Rl sites) and contains 13 bp at its 3' end that are identical with part of the consensus 60 bp repeat unit. Furthermore, this cDNA contains one SmaI (CCCGGG) site proximal to its 3' terminus. The SmaI site has been seen in all but one of the 60 bp repeat units analyzed to date and thus represents an accurate and convenient marker at which to locate the 3' part of the 5' cDNA sequence within the repeat unit itself. The nucleotide sequence shows that the longest open reading frame extends from an initiating methionine codon at nucleotide #58 through the 3' sequences that are identical with the consensus 60 bp repeat unit. Immediately preceding the putative ATG initiation codon is the nucleotide sequence CCACCACC that represents 2 perfect overlapping Kozak consensus (CCACC) initiation sequences (17). Downstream (7 amino acids) of the initiating methionine is a highly hydrophobic 13 a.a. peptide that includes 5 tandem leucine residues, that demonstrate preferred codon usage. Both because of its proximity to the amino terminus as well as its size it seems likely that this region represents a signal peptide directing the movement of the nascent protein into the lumen of the endoplasmic reticulum for subsequent secretion from the cell. Of further note is the high preponderance of serine residues - in one stretch of 20 amino acids (residues #43 to 62) the serine content is 40%. All these above features (i.e. longest ORF, Kozak consensus initiation sequences, location of signal peptide and preferred codon usage by leucine residues) make it highly probable that we are dealing with the correct reading frame.

The open reading frame extends into the 60 bp repeat unit and determines a proline rich 20 amino acid repeat motif that also contains 3 threonine, 2 serine, 2 glycine and 2-5 alanine residues. Due to nucleotide variations from the consensus sequence, the proline content within the repeat motif can vary, in which case alanine then substitutes for proline. The 20 a.a. repeat also contains histidine, valine, aspartic acid and arginine, whereas all other amino acids are not represented within the repeat motif.

Recombinant phages (psf7 and psf8) containing cDNA inserts corresponding to sequences 3' to the repeat array were obtained by

reprobing the cDNA library with unique genomic fragments located 3'
distal to the tandem repeats. The nucleotide sequences of psf7
(~1.8 kb) and psf 8 (1.6kb) show that they partially overlap and
whereas psf7 contains a number of repeat motifs and then extends 3'
beyond the repeat array, psf8 initiates approximately 200 bp downstream of the repeat array. Nucleotide sequencing of psf8 demonstrates that it is colinear with the genomic sequence (data not
shown). There is no evidence for any splicing events occurring in
the psf8 cDNA that corresponds to the 3' region of H23 Ag mRNA. The
psf 8 sequence extends the ORF 3' to the repeat array for an additional 160 a.a. at which point a TGA termination codon is encountered.
This is followed by a 3' untranslated region (UTR) of 1188 nucleotides.

As previously noted in the 5' sequence, the a.a. sequence 3' to
the repeat array is also very serine rich. Potential N-linked glycosylation sites (NXS/T) appear 4 times within this part of the protein
molecule and a hydrophobic region (VSFFFLSFHI) is located 48 amino
acids upstream of the carboxyl terminus. Although a poly A tail or
putative polyadenylation site has not been reached, the combined
length of the presented sequences 5' and 3' to the tandem array total
2.1 kb, which correlates well with previous estimates of the total
site of unique mRNA fragments.

The nucleotide sequence presented here thus probably corresponds
to an almost full length cDNA coding for the breast tumor associated
H23 antigen.

DISCUSSION

We have shown that a gene containing a variable number of tandem
repeats codes for an antigen detected by a monoclonal antibody, H23,
that was generated against particulate proteins secreted by breast
tumor cells.

Since the 225 bp 3b cDNA insert that codes only for the 20 amino
acid repeat motif was isolated by screening a gt11 cDNA expression
library with H23 MoAbs, it is highly probable that the actual epitope recognized by H23 MoAb is located within this repeat motif. Two
other groups have reported the isolation of monoclonal antibodies

(DF3, 2 and HMFG1 and HMFG2, 4) that although recognizing an epitope
situated within an almost identical 20 amino acid repeat motif (18,
19) do not differentiate between malignant and normal breast tissue.
Furthermore, the location of antigen detected by these "antimucin"
MoAbs is mostly apical compared to the intracellular location seen
in breast tumor tissue with our H23 MoAbs. We are thus faced with 2
apparent paradoxes.

A possible explanation of the first paradox may be that the
exact epitope recognized by "antimucin" MoAbs is different to that
detected by MoAbs (such as H23) which are preferentially tumor
specific. MoAbs specific for tumor tissue were generated against
either deglycosylated mucin i.e. core protein, (SM3, 11) or in our
case (H23), particulate proteins released by breast tumor cells (1).
It is possible that the tumor specific MoAbs are recognizing a non
glycosylated core protein epitope or a protein epitope glycosylated
differently to that produced in normal breast tissue. The "anti-
mucin" MoAbs may be recognizing a peptide epitope within the context
of a complex carbohydrate environment that is produced primarily in
normal epithelial tissue. Such MoAbs would thus have high affinity
for the glycosylated antigen made in normal epithelial tissues but
would also immune react with the differently processed antigen produced in breast tumor tissue. It has recently been demonstrated that
high molecular weight glycoproteins produced in breast tumor tissue
are differentially glycosylated compared with normal tissue,
supporting such an hypothesis (20).

In addition to its detection in breast tumor tissue, H23 Ag can
also be detected in the serum of breast cancer patients. The highly
hydrophobic 13 a.a. sequence situated 7 a.a. downstream of the putative initiating methionine conforms well to a signal peptide and
indicates that the H23 Ag mRNA probably codes for a secreted protein,
thus accounting for H23 Ag detection within the peripheral circulation as well as for apical localization.

It is more difficult to address the second paradox – that of the
intracellular location of H23 antigen detected in breast tumor
tissue. Two forms of antigen may possibly exist – one that is
primarily secreted whilst the other form, made in increased amounts

in the tumor tissue, is anchored within the cell. As the H23 MoAb recognizes intracellular as well as secreted antigen, we postulate that both these forms contain the 20 amino acid repeat motif. The 2 protein forms may differ in that the cellular located antigen has a transmembrane region, that anchors it to the cell. Such types of proteins are not without precedent, for example, immunoglobulins, major histocompatibility complex (MHC) antigens and neural cell adhesion molecules, N-CAMS (21-23). Indeed nucleotide sequencing of additional cDNA inserts corresponding to the region of mRNA 3' to the repeat array (λpsf7), indicates that differential splicing occurs here and may generate membrane-bound forms of the antigen. We are presently investigating whether this differentially spliced form of the H23 Ag mRNA is preferentially expressed in breast tumor tissue.

The full cDNA sequence presented here predicts that the final secreted antigen contains 287 amino acids besides those contributed by the 20 amino acid repeat motif. As the repeat array in any individual ranges from approximately 20 to 80 repeat units, each coding for the highly conserved 20 amino acids, the secreted antigen can contain 600 to 1800 amino acids. Every individual will have his or her own specific protein products that, because of size differences in the repeat motif, probably differ in their physicochemical characteristics. As it is likely that the antigen is somehow involved in the breast cancer process it is of obvious interest to see whether the clinical course of the disease correlates with a specific heterozygotic or homozygotic allelic configuration.

The full length cDNA sequence of the secreted antigen defines its amino acid sequence and allows us to prepare antibodies against peptides of the protein molecule other than those represented in the repeat motif itself. By using such an approach, greater specificity for breast tumor tissue may be obtained. Furthermore, as full length cDNA is now available, we can embark on experiments designed to elucidate the function of antigen in the tumorigenic process itself.

58

ACKNOWLEDGEMENTS

This work was supported by the Simko Chair for Breast Cancer Research, Frederico Fund for Tel Aviv University, grants from CNRS/ INSERM, Mr. Toby Green, London and the Israel Cancer Association (DHW). DHW, MH and IT were the recipients of EMBO Short Term Fellowships and DHW is the recipient of a Koret Foundation Fellow-ship, California. We thank Professor Pierre Chambon for continued support and fruitful discussions.

REFERENCES

1. Keydar, I., Chou, C.S., Hareuveni, M., Tsarfaty, I., Sahar, E., Seltzer, G., Chaitchik, S. and Hizi, A. Proc. Natl. Acad. Sci. U.S.A. 86 (4): 1362-1366, 1989.
2. Abe, M. and Kufe D. J. Cell. Physiol. 126: 126-136, 1976.
3. Bramwell, M.E., Bhavanandan, V.P., Wiseman, G. and Harris, H. Br. J. Cancer 48: 177-183, 1983.
4. Burchell, J.M., Durbin, H. and Taylor-Papadimitriou, J.J. Immunol. 131: 508-513, 1983.
5. Ceriani, R.L., Peterson, J.A. and Blank, E.W. Cancer Res. 44: 3033-3039, 1984.
6. Hilkens, J., Buijs, F., Hilgers, J., Hagemann, Ph., Calafat, J., Sonnenberg, A. and Van der Valk, M. Int. J. Cancer 34: 197-206, 1984.
7. Johnson, V.G., Schlom, J., Paterson, A.J., Bennett, J., Magnani, J.L. and Colcher, D. Cancer Res. 46: 850-857, 1986.
8. Lan, M.S., Finn, O.J., Fernsten, P.D. and Metzgar, R.S. Cancer Res. 45: 305-310, 1985.
9. Magnani, J.L., Steplewski, Z., Koprowski, H. and Ginsburg, V. Cancer Res. 43: 5489-5492, 1983.
10. Price, M.R., Edwards, S., Robins, R.A., Hilgers, J., Hilkens, J. and Baldwin, R. Eur. J. Can. Clin. Oncol. 22: 115-117, 1986.
11. Burchell, J., Gendler, S., Taylor-Papadimitrion, J., Girling, A. Lewis, A., Mills, R. and Lamport, D. Cancer Res. 47: 5476-5482, 1987.
12. Tsarfaty, I., Chaitchik, S., Hareuveni, M., Horev, J., Hizi, A., Wreschner, D.H. and Keydar, I. Monoclonal Antibodies and Breast Cancer San Francisco (in press), 1988.
13. Petkovitch, M., Brand, N.J., Krust, A. and Chambon, P. Nature 330: 445-450, 1987.
14. Sanger, F., Nicklen, S. and Coulson, A.R. Proc. Natl. Acad. Sci. U.S.A. 74: 5463-5467, 1977.
15. Jeffreys, A.J., Royle, N.J., Wilson, V. and Wong, Z. Nature 332: 278-281, 1988.
16. Nakamura, Y., Leppert, M., O'Connell, P., Wolff, R., Holm, T., Culver, M., Martin, C., Fujimoto, E., Hoff, M., Kumlin, E. and White, R. Science 235: 1616-1622, 1987.
17. Kozak, M. Cell 44: 283-292, 1986.

18. Siddiqui, J., Abe, M., Hayes, D., Shani, E., Yunis, E. and Kufe, D. Proc. Natl. Acad. Sci. U.S.A. 85: 2320-2323., 1988.
19. Gendler, S., Taylor-Papadimitrion, J., Duhig, T., Rothbard, J. and Burchell, J. J. Biol. Chem. 263: 12820-12823, 1988.
20. Rye, P.D. and Walker, R.A. Eur. J. Cancer Clin. Oncol. 25: 65-72, 1989.
21. Gough, N. Trends Genet. 3: 238-239, 1987.
22. Gussow, D. and Ploegh, H. Immunol. Today 8: 220-222, 1987.
23. Gower, H.S., Barton, C.H., Elson, V.L., Thompson, J., Moore, S.E., Dickson, G. and Walsh, F.S. Cell 55: 955-964, 1988.

5

EPITHELIAL MUCINS: EXPRESSION AND APPLICATIONS IN BREAST CANCER

M.R.PRICE, A.J.CLARKE and R.W.BALDWIN*

Cancer Research Campaign Laboratories, University of Nottingham,
Nottingham, NG7 2RD, U.K.

INTRODUCTION

A gene located in the 22 q region of the human chromosome 1
codes for a family of polymorphic, high molecular weight
glycoproteins which are associated with a variety of secretory
epithelia (1). Interest in these components stems largely from the
fact that they were found to be the target molecules for a whole
series of monoclonal antibodies, - produced independently in a
number of laboratories, - which were originally selected for
epithelial or breast tumour specificity (2,3). Compositional
analyses of purified antigen preparations demonstrated substantial
amounts of carbohydrate in O linkage to the serine and/or threonine
residues of the protein core via the sugar N-acetylgalactosamine.
This has led to their description as epithelial mucins.

MOLECULAR FEATURES OF EPITHELIAL MUCINS

Characterization of epithelial mucins with respect to their
detailed structure has not been rapid, and this is largely
attributable to their size (>400 kD) and complexity. However, the
recent demonstration that much of the protein core is encoded by a
tandem repeat of 60 bp has provided great insight into the nature of
these molecules (4-6). Variable numbers of the resulting 20 amino
acid repeated peptide in different individuals accounts for the

---

*Co-Chairman for Workshop: "Characterization and Follow-Up of Breast
Cancer Disease".

genetic polymorphism originally defined at the glycoprotein level (1,7,8). Furthermore, several of the anti-epithelial mucin monoclonal antibodies react with synthetic peptides corresponding to all or part of the predicted sequence of the 60 bp tandem repeat (5). For example, the C595 antibody, an IgG3 monoclonal antibody, prepared in our laboratories against affinity purified epithelial mucin, is inhibited in its binding to native epithelial antigen by pre-incubation with the 20 amino acid peptide. In addition, covalent linkage of the peptide to bovine serum albumin yields a conjugate to which the C595 antibody specifically binds.

The capacity to construct artificial immunoreactive conjugates using defined synthetic peptides clearly offers a new approach for producing novel monoclonal antibodies of known specificity for probing potential tumour associated epitopes in breast cancer. The finding that several antibodies have peptide epitopes also provides evidence that even in the fully processed mucin, the peptide core is accessible, at least in part, to allow antibody binding. Indeed, one antibody, the SM-3 antibody originally produced against chemically deglycosylated epithelial mucin from milk, preferentially reacts on histological sections with breast carcinomas and not benign mammary tumours or normal breast tissue (9). Hence, it is likely that in tumours, abberant glycosylation of mucins, resulting in increased accessibility of antibodies towards the protein core, may confer some antibodies with selective reactivity towards tumour-derived mucins. Alternatively, incomplete glycosylation or the action of tumour glycosyl transferases or glycosidases may generate novel epitopes preferentially found within tumours. These considerations will ultimately be a major influence in determining the clinical utility of antibodies against this family of molecules.

EXPRESSION OF EPITHELIAL MUCINS IN TUMOURS

In breast cancer, the gene encoding for the family of polymorphic epithelial mucins would appear to be virtually never switched off. Most breast carcinomas react to some degree with all the anti-mucin monoclonal antibodies although the type and extent

of staining of tissue sections may be of clinical relevance. The
tissue reactivity of the anti-breast carcinoma monoclonal antibody
NCRC-11, for example, has implications for prognosis since the
intensity of staining was found to be directly related to survival
(10,11). In independent, but more limited investigations by Angus
et al. (12), the tendency towards poorer prognosis for NCRC-11
negative tumours (i.e. containing less than 25% of positive cells)
failed to reach statistical significance, although it was
subsequently determined that NCRC-11 staining showed a negative
correlation with epidermal growth factor receptor status (13), this
being regarded as an indicator of poor prognosis (14).

In normal breast tissue, NCRC-11 staining predominates at the
luminal surfaces of ducts and acini. This expression of epithelial
mucins is consistent with their association with the membranes of
exfoliated or secreted milk fat globules. In tumours, there is a
loss in this functional cellular polarity, which together with
disruption of tissue architecture by the developing tumour,
facilitates access of tumour-derived mucins to the circulation.
This therefore represents one mechanism by which epithelial mucin,
either from the tumour itself or possibly from disrupted normal
epithelia adjacent to the tumour, may become a circulating marker
indicative of progressive disease. The measurement of these markers
and assessment of their relevance in breast cancer has become a
central topic of investigation.

EPITHELIAL MUCINS AS CIRCULATING TUMOUR MARKERS

Circulating mucins are elevated in breast cancer patients in
comparison to the normal healthy control subjects (reviewed in
15,16). This has been established using double determinant or
two-site radioimmunometric assays (sandwich immunoassays) employing
single or combinations of monoclonal antibodies. Since many
epitopes of tumour-associated epithelial mucins are repeated
structures, then a single monoclonal antibody may be used both to
capture antigen from the serum sample and subsequently to detect the
captured antigen using a radioisotope or ELISA-based system for

quantitation (homologous double determinant immunoassays). The combination of two different antibodies (in heterologous double determinant immunoassays) permits serum antigens to be captured and then detected by separate epitopes.

In homologous immunoassays, elevated levels of circulating mucins have been detected in breast cancer patients using the anti-milk fat globule membrane antibodies HMFG-1 and HMFG-2 (17). 115D8 (18,19) and W1 (20) and also in tests using the anti-tumour antibodies NCRC-11 (21); DF-3 (22) and 3E1.2 (23). Heterologous immunoassays have been developed using various combinations of antibodies such as 115D8 + DF3 (15), BC4E 549 and BC4N 154 (24) M29 + M38 (20), and even polyclonal and monoclonal antibodies have been brought together, in the same immunoassay (25). The sensitivity for the detection of elevated antigen levels in breast cancer patients is variously reported from around 30% up to 90%. Direct comparisons are, however, difficult since the choice of individuals in both the patient groups and the group comprising the normal controls varies between investigations.

In initial studies using the NCRC-11 antibody in an homologous assay system, over 40% of patients with advanced breast cancer showed elevated levels of circulating antigen (21). Subsequent tests confirmed this level of sensitivity and also demonstrated that only about 2% of patients with benign breast disease were elevated with respect to serum NCRC-11 antigen. Mean antigen levels in clinically stratified patient groups tended to increase with increasing extent and severity of disease (26).

The question as to why only a proportion of breast cancer patients have elevated serum antigen levels has been considered by Tjandra et al. (27). Their assay, based upon the use of the antibody 3E1.2 which reacts with a high molecular weight antigen termed Mammary Serum Antigen (MSA - 23), detected elevated antigen levels in about 70% of patients with localized breast cancer and in about 90% of patients with advanced disease. To determine if there were any special immunohistological features of subjects with normal or raised MSA levels, a retrospective study of patients with Stage I (node negative) breast cancer was conducted (27). The preliminary findings suggested that the MSA level in localized breast cancer was related particularly to the degree of immunoperoxidase staining with antibody 3E1.2, to tumour size, and weakly with tumour grade. Clearly, these findings require further investigation since, as with the studies with the NCRC-11 antibody (10,11), it appears that immunohistological staining of tumour tissues may provide information relating to prognosis.

EPITHELIAL MUCINS VS. CEA IN BREAST CANCER

Carcinoembryonic antigen (CEA) is the most widely used marker for monitoring the clinical course of patients with breast cancer although its applications are limited by poor sensitivity. Comparison of the results of measuring circulating epithelial mucins with the assay of serum CEA has revealed that elevated marker levels are more frequently associated with mucin determinations and that there is no correlation between levels of the two types of marker. It also appears that the additive effect of measuring epithelial mucins and CEA may only be marginally better than for the mucins alone since CEA only becomes informative as a tumour marker in a fraction of patients whose disease has disseminated (28,29).

EPITHELIAL MUCINS FOR MONITORING BREAST CANCER

Several investigations have now shown that measurement of circulating epithelial mucins provides information of potential clinical utility. This is exemplified in a comparative study of circulating NCRC-11 antigen and CEA which were measured in sequential serum samples from 37 patients undergoing therapy for breast cancer (30). At least 4 serum samples were collected from each patient over a mean period of study of 5 months. From the individual measurements of each patient, a linear regression analysis was used to calculate a mean change in antigen level per month over the time during which samples were taken for each patient. These measurements were then related to the independent clinical assessments of the course of disease. In Table 1 it is evident that in the group of patients with progressive disease, both NCRC-11 antigen levels, and less prominently, CEA levels, were

Table 1: - Changing serum antigen levels related to patient classification according to course of disease

Patient Grouping According To The Course of Disease	NCRC-11 Antigen		CEA (ng/ml)	
	Unit change per month (Mean $\pm$ SD)	Range	Unit change per month (Mean $\pm$ SD)	Range
Progressor (n = 14)	19 ± 23^1	$-18 \rightarrow 54$	2.2 ± 4.9^2	$-2.9 \rightarrow 15.1$
Stable (n = 11)	-11 ± 46	$-124 \rightarrow 26$	-0.1 ± 0.4	$-0.9 \rightarrow 0.3$
Responder (n = 12)	-22 ± 18	$-46 \rightarrow 0$	-1.0 ± 2.5	$-8.1 \rightarrow 0.2$

[1] - NCRC-11 serum antigen values in the Progressor Group were significantly different (P<0.01) from those in the Stable and Responder Groups.

[2] - The comparison between the Progressor and Responder Groups with respect to changes in CEA levels, was the only comparison to approach statistical significance (P<0.05).

increasing. Patients with stable disease and responding disease showed decreasing marker levels and the differences between these groups and the progressor group were more pronounced with respect to measurements of NCRC-11 antigen (Table 1).

The sensitivity of this procedure for descriminating between the three groups of patients was investigated and the findings are shown in Table 2. Measurements of NCRC-11 antigen more accurately identified patients with stable and responding disease as compared to patients with progressive disease (73% and 75% cf. 57%, respectively). CEA determinations were insensitive to disease progression or response. Increases or decreases in either NCRC-11 serum antigen or CEA were highly specific for disease progression or response, respectively (Table 2). However, a lack of serum marker movement was much less specific for identifying the group of patients with stable disease (65% specificity for NCRC-11 and only 23% specificity for CEA, for identifying Stable patients - Table 2). The present findings would therefore suggest that the NCRC-11 serum antigen assay may have a role in monitoring cancer therapy and that this assay is considerably more informative than CEA determination.

Table 2: - Analysis of the changes in NCRC-11 antigen and CEA levels with respect to their capacity to monitor the clinical course of disease

Assay Performance Parameter	Serum Marker Assay	
	NCRC-11 Antigen	CEA
Sensitivity[1] of Assay for Identifying:		
Progressive Disease	8/14 (57%)	3/14 (21%)
Stable Disease	8/11 (73%)	11/11 (100%)
Responding Disease	9/12 (75%)	2/10 (20%)
Specificity of Assay for Defining:		
Progressive Disease [2]	22/23 (96%	23/23 (100%)
Stable Disease [3]	17/26 (65%)	6/26 (23%)
Responding Disease [4]	22/25 (88%)	24/25 (96%)

[1] - Sensitivity of assay for defining a condition
= [No. with condition and identified accurately by marker assay]
÷ [Total No. with condition]

[2] - Specificity of marker assay for defining Progressive Disease
= [No. identified as Responders + No. identified as Stable]
÷ [No. in Responder Group + No. in Stable Group]

[3] - Specificity of marker assay for defining Stable Disease
= [No. identified as Progressors + No. identified as Responders]
÷ [No. in Progressor Group + No. in Responder Group]

[4] - Specificity of marker assay for defining Responding Disease
= [No. identified as Progressors + No. identified as Stable]
÷ [No. in Progressor Group + No. in Stable Group]

CONCLUSION

Even though epithelial mucins are products of normal, as well as malignant cells, they have much to commend themselves as tumour markers in breast cancer. Immunoassays, based upon the use of the presently available monoclonal antibodies, most accurately reflect clinical changes in patients with disseminated disease. However, advances in defining the structure of epithelial mucins will lead to an understanding of the subtle molecular features by which tumour-derived mucins can be distinguished from their normal cell counterparts. With such knowledge, it is anticipated that new, second generation monoclonal antibodies will be produced with greater selective reactivity for breast cancer.

ACKNOWLEDGEMENTS

These studies were supported by the Cancer Research Campaign and by the XOMA Corporation, California.

REFERENCES

1. Swallow, D.M., Gendler, S., Griffiths, B., Corney, G., Taylor-Papadimitriou, J. and Bramwell, M. Nature, 327: 82-84, 1987.
2. Price, M.R. In: Subcellular Biochemistry, Vol.12, Immunological Aspects, (Ed. J.R. Harris), Plenum Press, London. 1988, pp. 1-30.
3. Price, M.R. Eur.J.Clin.Oncol., 24: 1700-1804, 1988.
4. Gendler, S.J., Burchell, J., Duhig, T., White, R., Parker, M. and Taylor-Papadimitriou, J. Proc. Natl. Acad. Sci. USA, 84: 6060-6064, 1987.
5. Gendler, S., Taylor-Papadimitriou, J., Duhig, T., Rothbard, J. and Burchell, J. J. Biol. Chem., 263: 12820-12823, 1988.
6. Siddiqui, J., Abe, M., Hayes, D., Shani, E., Yunis, E. and Kufe, D. Proc. Natl. Acad. Sci. USA., 85: 2320-2323, 1988.
7. Karlsson, S., Swallow, D.M., Griffiths, R., Corney, G., Hopkinson, D.A., Dawney, A. and Carton, J.P. Ann. Hum. Genet., 47: 263-269, 1983.
8. Swallow, D.M., Griffiths, B., Bramwell, M., Wiseman, G. and Burchell, J. Disease Markers, 4: 247-254, 1986.
9. Burchell, J., Gendler, S., Taylor-Papadimitriou, J., Girling, A., Lewis, A., Millis, R. and Lamport, D. Cancer Res., 47: 5476-5482, 1987.
10. Ellis, I.O., Hinton, C.P., MacNay, J., Robins, R.A., Elston, C.W., Owainati, A., Blamey, R.W., Baldwin, R.W. and Ferry, B. Br. Med. J., 290: 881-883, 1985.
11. Ellis, I.O., Bell, J., Todd, J.M., Williams, M., Dowle, C., Robins, R.A., Elston, C.W., Blamey, R.W. and Baldwin, R.W. Br. J. Cancer, 56: 295-300, 1987.
12. Angus, B., Napier, J. and Purvies, J. J. Pathol., 149: 301-306, 1986.
13. Wright,C., Angus, B., Napier, J., Wetherall, M., Udagawa, Y., Sainsbury, J.R.C., Johnston, S., Carpenter, F. and Horne, C.H.W. J. Pathol., 153: 325-331, 1987.
14. Sainsbury, J.R.C., Malcolm, A.J., Appleton, D.R., Farndon, J.R. and Harris, A.L. J. Clin. Pathol., 38: 1225-1228, 1985.
15. Kufe, D., Hayes, D. and Abe, M. In: Cancer Diagnosis In Vitro Using Monoclonal Antibodies (Ed. Kupchick, H.Z.,) Immunology Series Volume 39, M. Dekker, New York, 1988, pp 67-100.

16. Kenemans, P., Bast, R.C., Yemeda, C.A., Price, M.R. and Hilgers, J. In: Cancer Reviews (Eds, J. Hilgers and S. Zotter), Vol.11, Munksgaard, 1989, In press.
17. Burchell, J., Wang, D. and Taylor-Papadimitriou, J. Int. J. Cancer, 34: 763-768, 1984.
18. Hilkens, J., Kroezen, V., Bonfrer, J.M.G., De Jong-Bakker, M. and Bruning, P.F. Cancer Res., 46: 2582-2587, 1986.
19. Hilkens, J., Bonfrer, J.M.G., Kroezen, V., Van Eykeren, M., Nooyen, W., De Jong Bakker, M. and Bruning, P.F. Int. J. Cancer, 39: 431-435, 1987.
20. Linsley, P.S., Brown, J.P., Magnani, J.P. and Namer, M. Br. J. Cancer, 55: 567-569, 1987.
21. Price, M.R., Crocker, G., Edwards, S., Nagra, I.S., Robins, R.A., Williams, M., Blamey, R.W., Swallow, D.M. and Baldwin, R.W. Eur. J. Cancer Clin. Oncol., 23: 1169-1176, 1987.
22. Hayes, D.F., Sekine, H., Ohno, T., Abe, M., Keefe, K. and Kufe, D.W. J. Clin. Invest., 75: 1671-1678, 1985.
23. Stacher, S.A., Sacks, N.P.M., Golder, J., Tjandra, J.J., Thompson, C.H., Smithyman, A. and McKenzie, I.F.C. Br. J. Cancer, 57: 298-303, 1988.
24. Bray, K.R., Koda, J.E. and Gaur, P.K. Cancer Res., 47: 5853-5860, 1987.
25. Ashorn, P., Kallioniemi, O.-P., Hietanen, T., Ashorn, R. and Krohn, K. Int. J. Cancer, Suppl.2: 28-33, 1988.
26. Robertson, J.F.R., Price, M.R., Selby, C., Pearson, D., Ellis, I.O. and Blamey, R.W. Br. J. Surg., Abstract, In press, 1989.
27. Tjandra, J.J., Busmanis, I., Russell, I.S., Collins, R.G., Reed, R.G. and McKenzie, I.F.C. Br. J. Cancer, 58: 815-817, 1988.
28. Pons-Anicet, D.M.F., Krebs, B.P., Mira, R. and Namer, M. Br. J. Cancer, 55: 567-569, 1987.
29. Tondini, C., Hayes, D.F., Gelman, R., Henderson, I.C. and Kufe, D.W. Cancer Res., 48: 4107-4112, 1988.
30. Price, M.R., Clarke, A.J., Robertson, J.F.R., Baldwin, R.W. and Blamey, R.W. Br. J. Cancer, submitted, 1989.

6

BREAST CANCER DETECTION, DIAGNOSIS, AND RADIATION THERAPY
Daniel B. Kopans, M.D.

Department of Radiology Massachusetts General Hospital,

and Harvard Medical School Boston, Massachusetts 02114

The fact that there has been little change in the
mortality from breast cancer in the past 60 years has
resulted in an evolution in the approach to detection,
diagnosis, and therapy. The refinement in mammographic
techniques, and improvement in resolution has resulted in
the ability to detect more breast cancers at an earlier
stage than in the past. By recognizing that breast
cancer does not follow the Halstedian concept of an
orderly direct extension and spread from the breast along
the lymphatics to the rest of the body the approach to
treatment now addresses the frequently disparate problems
of local, regional, and systemic control. Until host
immune responses are better understood and used to
interrupt the progression of the disease, or until its
etiologies are defined, and preventive methods elucidated
the only significant impact on mortality appears to be
earlier detection. Despite the greatest scrutiny there
are stiil numerous controversies surrounding breast
cancer detection, diagnosis, and therapy, and these are
likely to persist until the basic biology of this
spectrum of diseases is better understood.

In the 1960's a prospective randomized, controled

study of breast cancer screening was undertaken within
The Health Insurance Plan of New York (HIP) (1). The
62,000 women age 40-65 within the plan were randomized to
a study group that was offered physical examination and
mammography annually for 4 years and a control group of
31,000 women who were not informed of the study and had
routine health care. The trial was designed to answer
the question - Can screening beginning at age 40 reduce
the mortality from breast cancer. Despite the fact that
30% of the study group never attended a screen there were
20-25% fewer deaths from breast cancer in the study
group, and this benefit has lasted beyond 18 years. By
using a randomized controlled study and death as the
measured end point the HIP results as well as the more
recent Swedish data eliminate the often cited concerns of
lead time bias, and length bias sampling. Furthermore,
the population based randomized, controlled Swedish study
in the 1970's (2) used only mammography to screen women
40-74, and by demonstrating a similar 30% mortality
reduction established the validity of mammography for
screening. These results lend greater credence to the
retrospective comparisons of the Breast Cancer Detection
Demonstration project (BCDDP) data to mortality rates
monitored in the Surveillance, Epidemiology and End
Results (SEER) program in the United States (3,4) which
clearly demonstrated the ability of mammography to detect
breast cancer at an earlier stage and produce a

commensurate reduction in breast cancer deaths. Similar, and even greater mortality reduction was found in case control studies in the Netherlands (5,6). Analysis of the Swedish data suggests that the reduction in mortality from mammographic screening is due to a shift toward earlier stage lesions at the time of diagnosis (7).

Despite the preponderance of data in support of screening, controversy persists. It is likely that much of the argument is due to the anticipated economic costs of breast cancer screening. For example, PAP screening for cervical cancer has been universally adopted despite the lack of data from randomized controlled trials to prove its efficacy. Its relatively low cost has not made it the focus of health planners despite a study in the Netherlands showing that from a cost/benefit point of view mammographic screening is more efficacious than PAP testing due to the much greater prevalence of breast cancer (8).

Much of the controversy centers around the question of who should be screened, and at what interval. Arguments arose when the data in the screening programs were, retrospectively, stratified by age. Despite the fact that the studies were not originally designed with sufficient power to permit this, analyses have, nevertheless, been done, and the early reviews failed to show a statistically significant reduction in mortality for women 40-49. More recent analyses have shown that

the mortality reduction for women over 50 occurred soon
after the onset of screening while benefit was delayed by
6-7 years for younger women. Chu et al have recently
reviewed the HIP data examining only women with breast
cancer, and have shown a statistically significant
reduction in mortality for women 40-49 that did not begin
to occur until six years after the start of the study
(9).

In order to reduce the number of women who should be
screened it might initially seem reasonable to screen
only women in high risk categories. The baseline risk in
the United States for women who are not at elevated risk
of developing breast cancer is 4-5%. Factors such as
early menarche, late menopause, late or nulliparity, and
a family history of breast cancer have been shown to
increase the chances of developing breast cancer so that
the combined risk for all American women has been
estimated by the American Cancer Society at 10%. Since
by far the greatest risks for developing breast cancer
are gender and age it is not surprising that 75% of
breast cancers occur in women with none of the other
associated risks (10). It has been estimated that only
25% of breast cancers occur in women with additional risk
beyond that of gender and age. Thus, if screening were
confined to only women with elevated risk 75% of the
cancers would avoid early detection. Since it is not yet
possible to predict who will develop breast cancer, who

is protected from breast cancer, or how to prevent breast
cancer all women must be considered at risk and should
have access to screening.

In 1983 the American Cancer Society issued guidelines
for breast cancer screening. These suggested:

    1. A mammogram every 1 or 2 years age 40-49

    2. Annual mammography after age 50

These guidelines were based on the best estimates of
benefit prior to that time. The United States National
Cancer Institute has recently adopted and supported the
ACS guidelines although screening women 40-49 remains
controversial (11).

More recent data suggest that in fact the guidelines
are inverted. It appears that women age 40-49 should be
screened on a more frequent, annual schedule and as data
accumulate they suggest that it may be possible to extend
the interval for women over 50. The basis for this
apparent reversal and more aggressive approach in younger
women was first proposed by Moskowitz in his analysis of
women screened in the Cincinnati BCDDP (12) and recently
corroborated by the screening data from Sweden (13). It
appears that the lead time gained by mammographic
screening in women 40-49 is shorter than for women over
50 and thus the interval between screens must be shorter
to maximize the benefit. Mammography appears to be able
to detect breast cancer, on average 3.0 to 4 years before
it is palpable in women age 50 and over while this "lead

time" is reduced to 2 to 2.5 years for women 40-49. Thus if one were to screen women 40-49 every 2 years little advantage would accrue over physical examination. This may explain the lack of mortality reduction in the Swedish screening program for women age 40-49 who were screened every 2 years. The Breast Imaging Committee of the American College of Radiology has unanimously agreed that a shorter interval between screens (annual) should be instituted for women 40-49. Adoption of this modification in the guidelines has been delayed by other American groups due to political concerns. Recognition in Sweden of the importance of a shorter interval for "younger" women has led to the adoption of a more aggressive screening program for women 40-49 using two view mammography rather than the single view, lower sensitivity method originally used in the two county study.

Recently, new controversy has arisen from the early data published from a second Swedish screening program in Malmo (14). Although the screened population should ultimately demonstrate a benefit from screening since there was a trend toward earlier stage lesions in the study population this is not yet apparent in the early data. These are likely too preliminary to make firm assessment and the statistical power of the study appears to be insufficient give the number of women enrolled. Further complicating the Malmo study is the fact that 24%

of the control group underwent mammography, and 20% of the cancers in the control group were detected by mammography. Thus the power of the Malmo study is severely diluted and compromised. An additional trial whose data will be forthcoming is in Canada comparing the effect of screening by physical examination with mammographic screening. Unfortunately the data from that study will be difficult to interpret due to the poor quality of the mammography in the early years of the trial.

Based on the data presently available, and the quality of the data that will be forthcoming the best medical advice for women is listed below. These health guidelines will be modified by government planners to address the issues of cost. For example, if immediate benefit is sought, then screening only women 50 and over will be supported since the benefit for younger women will be delayed by 5-10 years.

PROJECTED GUIDELINES

    1. Annual mammography beginning at age 40

    2. Possible longer screening interval after 50
       (18-24 months)

The greatest impediment to mammographic screening will be cost. This must be balanced against the need for accuracy. The highest imaging quality is required in a screening program since this is the only chance one might have to detect the lesion earlier. Centers dedicated to high quality screening permit efficient imaging. In an effort to minimize cost, batch interpretation will become the norm (15). Women requiring additional evaluation due to a sign or symptom of breast cancer, or a question raised on screening will return to a diagnostic center where an on-site radiologist will monitor additional views and perform ultrasound, aspiration, and localization procedures. Association of screening centers with diagnostic and therapeutic centers will improve the continuity of care and help support a woman through an anxiety provoking period.

Since mammography misses 10% of cancers that are palpable, screening should include a physical examination, and two view mammography. The standard views are a mediolateral and craniocaudal projection of both breasts. The mediolateral/oblique usually maximizes the tissue projected onto the detector, and is preferred. If patients are referred by a physician, the physical examination should be performed by the referring doctor. If self-referred women are accepted a physical examination should be offered by the center, or at the least the woman should be informed of the need for physical examination as well. Based on the number of cancers that are detected by women between screens it is likely that screening by both physical examination and mammography on an annual basis will not detect 20% of cancers. This should be made clear to women so that they do not delay seeking diagnosis if a mass appears between screens. Furthermore, it should be clearly understood that no test or combination of tests can exclude breast cancer. The role of screening is not to exclude cancer, but to detect it earlier and improve the chances for longer term survival.

Mammography detects many lesions that are not cancer, but must be differentiated from cancer. In organized screening programs the predictive value of mammography ranges from 50-70% due to the relatively stable population (16). However, until a population based screening program is instituted with good compliance, and repetitive screening of the same women, the predictive value for mamography is likely to be high (17,18,19). Compounding the issue is the medicolegal climate in some countries where "failure to diagnose" breast cancer without delay leads to excessive biopsies. Regardless, accurate guidance for the surgeon to non-palpable lesions is required to insure safe, and accurate diagnosis and removal of clinically occult lesions. A haphazard approach to these lesions should be discouraged. Many techniques have been described to permit aggressive diagnosis by permitting safe and accurate guidance for the surgeon (20,21,22,23,24,25,26).

The advantage of earlier detection lies not only in

reduced mortality, but in the greater therapeutic options available including so called conservation therapy with surgical excision, and radiation to eliminate any residual, clinically inapparent foci of cancer.

It is beyond the scope of this review to address all the issues involved in breast cancer therapy. However, concurrent with the demonstration of the importance of earlier diagnosis in breast cancer has been the demonstration that management and control of cancer in the breast does not require the extensive surgery once thought to be necessary. Furthermore, the ability to diagnose breast cancer earlier makes conservation therapy more likely to be cosmetically successful. Recognition that cancer can spread not only by contiguity, but as emboli along vascular and lymphatic routes has resulted in therapeutic approaches that address the separate issues involved in local, regional, and systemic control. It has been shown that one mode of therapy is unlikely to be successful in controlling tumor in all areas. By recognizing that overall survival does not merely depend on eradicating the primary tumor in the breast several large studies have confirmed the approach now accepted by modern therapists of treating the breast as a problem of local control and attacking the probability of distant spread as a separate problem requiring a systemic approach. The demonstration that radical surgery was not needed permitted a "conserving" approach to the breast itself that is more acceptable to many women. Prospective trials including those from Milan (27), the National Surgical Adjuvant breast project (NSABP) in the United States (28), and the Institut Gustave-Roussy in France (29) as well as retrospective reviews have demonstrated that tumor removal with a margin of normal breast followed by supervoltage radiation therapy with a boost to the tumor bed for a total of 5000 to 7000 cGy has the same probability of local control as the more mutilating mastectomy. The risk of local recurrence in the conservation patients at 5 years was under 10% and comparable to mastectomy, and failure in the preserved breast appears to be more successfully treated than a chest wall failure following mastectomy. To date overall survival appears similar.

Despite the vast amount of research on breast cancer therapy is a remarkably poor understanding of the development and progression of these malignancies. There is still heated debate concerning the relationship of in-situ forms of breast cancer to the lethal invasive lesion. As more studies evolve it has become apparent that there are numerous factors that set of one tumor from another, and our crude staging methods will likely undergo subdivisions as more prognostic factors are recognized and dictate differing therapeutic approaches. Host responses likely are the ultimate determinant of treatment success or failure, and a greater understanding of these complex issues will permit more accurate targeting of therapy.

Breast cancer has unique psycho-social aspects that must be considered in therapeutic decisions, and these have stimulated the present focus on breast preservation. There is the possibility that new emerging data may reverse this trend in some situations. As greater understanding of growth factors evolves, along with an understanding of the interrelationship of breast tissue and the possible nurturing of metastatic disease by factors elaborated by the remaining breast tissue the pendulum may swing again. At this time the data support an approach that combines surgery, and radiation therapy with a boost to the tumor bed for local control, and the use of chemotherapy and hormonal manipulation to address the problem of systemic spread. Ultimately a better understanding of the etiologies and natural history of breast cancer will permit more targeted therapy that recognizes each individual situation, and ultimately prevents the initiation or promotion sequences.

REFERENCES

1. Shapiro S; Venet W; Venet L; and Roeser R. Ten to Fourteen-Year Effect of Screening on Breast Cancer Mortality. Journal of the National Cancer Institute. (1982) 69 No.2:349-355.

2. Tabar L; Fagerberg CJG; Gad A; Baldetorp L; Holmberg LH; Grontoft O; Ljungquist U; Lundstrom B; and Manson JC. Reduction in Mortality from Breast Cancer after Mass Screening with Mammography. Lancet. (1985) 1:829-832.

3. Seidman H; Gelb SK; Silverberg E; LaVerda N; and Lubera JA. Survival Experience in the Breast Cancer Detection Demonstration Project. Ca-A Cancer Journal for Clinicians. (1987) 37 No. 5:258-290.

4. Morrison AS, Brisson J, Khalid N. Breast Cancer Incidence and Mortality in th Breast Cancer Detection Demonstration Project. JNCI 1988, Vol. 80: No. 19:17-24.

5. Verbeek ALM; Hendriks JHCL; Holland R; Mravunac M; Sturmans F; and Day NE. Reduction of Breast Cancer Mortality Through Mass Screening with Modern. Mammography. Lancet. (1984) June 2:1222-1224.

6. Collette HJA; Day NE; Rombach JJ; and DeWaard F. Evaluation of Screening for Breast Cancer in a Non-Randomized Study (The Dom Project) by means of a Case-Control Study. Lancet. (1984) June 2:1224-1226.

7. Tabar L; Duffy SW; and Krusemo UB. Detection Method, Tumor Size and Node Metastases in Breast Cancers Diagnosed During a Trial of Breast Cancer Screening. Eur J Cancer Clin Oncol. (1987) 23 No.7:959-962.

8. International Workshop on Information Systems in Breast Cancer Detection. National Cancer Institute and the FDA. Rockville Maryland Dec. 8-10, 1988.

9. Chu KC, Smart CR, Tarone RE. Analysis of Breast Cancer Mortality and Stage Distribution by Age for the Health Insurance Plan Clinical Trial. JNCI Vol. 80, No. 14. September 21, 1988 1125-1132

10. Seidman H, Stellman SD, and Mushinski MH.A Different Perspective on Breast Cancer Risk Factors: Some Implications of Nonattributable Risk. Cancer. 1982 Vol.32 No.5:301-313.

11. Eddy DM; Hasselblad V; McGivney W; and Hendee W. The Value of Mammography Screening in Women Under 50 Years. JAMA. (1988) 259 No.10:1512-1549.

12. Moskowitz M. Breast Cancer: Age-Specific Growth Rates and Screening Strategies. Rad. (1986) 161:37-41.

13. Tabar L, Faberberg G, Day NE, Holmberg L. What is the Optimum Interval Between Mammographic Screening Examinations? - An Analysis Based on the Latest Results of the Swedish Two-county Breast Screening Trial. Br. J. Cancer 19897, 55:547-551

14. Andersson I, Aspegren K, Janzon L, Landberg T, Lindholm K, et al. Mammographic Screening and Mortality from Breast Cancer: The Malmo Mammographic Screening Trial. BMJ 1988; 297:943-949.

15. Sickles EA; Weber WN; Galvin HB; Ominsky SH; and Sollitto RA. Mammographic Screening: How to Operate

Successfully at Low Cost. Rad. (1986) 160:95-97.
16. Kopans DB, Swann CA. Observations on Mammographic Screening and False-Positive Mammograms. AJR 1988, 150:785-786
17. Gisvold JJ, & Martin JK, Prebiopsy Localization of Nonpalpable Breast Lesions. AJR 1984;143: 477-481
18. Meyer JE, Kopans DB, Stomper PC, and Lindfors KK. Occult Breast Abnormalities:Percutaneous Precperative Needle Localization. Rad. 1984, 150:335-337.
19. Rosenberg AL, Schwartz GF, Feig SA, and Patchefsky AS. Clinically Occult Breast Lesions: Localization and Significance. Rad. 1987, 162:167-170.
20. Kopans DB, and Meyer JE. The Versatile Spring-Hookwire Breast Lesion Localizer.AJR. 1982, 138:586-587. springhook
21. Kopans DB, Meyer JE, Lindfors KK, and McCarthy KA. Spring-Hookwire Breast Lesion Localizer: Use with Rigid Compression Mammographic Systems. Rad. 1985, 157:505-507.

22. Kopans DB, and Meyer JE. Computed Tomography Guided Localization of Clinically Occult Breast Carcinoma - The "N" Skin Guide. Rad. 1982, 145:211-212.
23. Kopans DB, Meyer JE, Lindfors KK, and Bucchianeri SS. Breast Sonography to Guide Aspiration of Cysts and Preoperative Localization of Occult Breast Lesions. AJR. 1984, 143:489-492.
24. Swann CA, Kopans DB, McCarthy KA, White G, and Hall DA. Occult Breast Lesions:Practical Solutions to Problems of Triangulation and Localization. Rad. 1987;163:577-579.
25. Kopans DB, Waitzkin ED, Linetsky L, Swann CA, McCarthy KA, Hall DA, and White G. Localization of Breast Lesions Identified on Only One Mammographic View. AJR. 1987, 149:39-41.
26. Kopans DB, Swann CA. Preoperative Imaging-Guided Needle Placement and Localization of Clinically Occult Breast Lesions. AJR 1989;152:1-9
27. Veronisi U: Randomized Trials Comparing Conservatio Techniques with Conventional Surgery: An Overview. In Tobias JS, Peckham MJ (Eds): Primary management of Breast Cancer: Alternatives to Mastectomy Management of malignant Disease Series, pp 131-152. London, E. Arnold 1985.
28. Fisher B, Bauer M., Margolese R, et al: Five Year Results of a Randomized Clinical Trial Comparing Total Mastectomy and Segmental Mastectomy with or without Radiation in the Treatment of Breast Cancer. N. Engl J Med 312:665, 1985.
29. Sarazin D, Le M, Rouesse J, et al: Conservative Treatment Versus Mastectomy in Breast Cancer tumors with Microscopic Diameter of 20 mm. or less. Cancer 53:1209, 1984.

7

SURGICAL STRATEGIES IN CURABLE BREAST CANCER

R. ROZIN

INTRODUCTION

There is a lack of uniformity governing the surgical treatment of curable breast carcinoma. For almost 80 years there was a rigid uniform policy of treatment for curable cancer - the radical mastectomy procedure. During that time there were some rebels who disagreed with the dominant opinions and methods of treatment. In their time they were considered heretics but later became pioneers of a new approach to curable breast cancer.

There is a proper operation for each stage of the disease, but we lack accurate information regarding the exact extent of the disease. If the extent of the disease were known precisely, then we could choose with certainty the scope of the operation.

For cancers in other regions of the body, as in carcinoma of the stomach, the colon or liver, we readily employ the most extensive operation which does not endanger the life of the patient, in order to radically remove the tumor, its lymphatic drainage, and the entire regional lymph gland system. When it applies to the breast, this becomes unacceptable. Estetic and psychological considerations have created constant pressure on the surgical community to reduce the scope of the operation so as not to remove the breast and inflict psychological damage on the woman.

A SHORT SURGICAL HISTORY

Radical mastectomy, which involves the removal of the breast, the pectoralis major muscle and the regional lymph nodes, became standard in the 1890s. During the first decades of this century

the surgical world concentrated on enlarging the scope of radical
mastectomy in search of procedures which would improve cure rates
and lessen local recurrence. Many years later, it became evident
that extending the resection beyond the axilla to the supra-
clavicular region and to under the sternum only increased morbidity
without significantly increasing survival.

In the middle of the century, the heretics pulled to the
opposite direction by attempting to define the smallest surgical
procedure which would obtain the same results as radical mastectomy.

We are now in the midst of trials to define the frontiers of
minimal surgery. Had prospective randomized studies been started
many years ago, we probably could today define optimal surgery.
It takes ten to 20 years of following up many hundreds of women
with the same stage of disease, receiving identical treatment,
before we can evaluate any treatment modality. Extensive cooperative studies of this kind have only been undertaken during the
last few decades, notably those headed by Dr. Bernard Fisher and
by Dr. Umberto Veronesi.

The mortality rate, that is the death per 100,000 population,
has not changed significantly in the past 50 years. Variations in
surgery and/or radiotherapy have failed to have a significant
impact on the mortality rate.

There has been some improvement in the relative 5 year
survival rate in the past decades. When patients are compared
stage for stage this must be viewed with caution in light of the
continuing stability of the mortality rate. The improvement may be
due in part to the detection of more cancers in their localized
and preclinical stages. Some lesions classified as breast cancer
may look malignant histologically but biologically behave in a
benign fashion.

FROM BIOPSY TO SURGERY

Breast Biopsy is required to determine the malignant nature of a
breast abnormality. A few methods are available:

Excision biopsy: Excision biopsy is preferable. The pathologist can select representative areas for microscopic studies and

for estrogen receptor studies.

Incision biopsy: This is useful to confirm the diagnosis in advanced cancer. It helps confirm the benign nature of a large fibrocystic breast area.

Fine needle biopsy: Needle biopsy requires a very good cytologist. The sensitivity – meaning the probability that the test will be positive when cancer is present – varies from 74-96%. A negative cytological report must not be accepted for a dominant solid mass and open biopsy should follow.

The specificity of fine needle aspiration – meaning the probability that the test will be negative when cancer is absent – varies from 79-100%.

Core needle has from 67-90% sensitivity. The accuracy is related to the tumor size.

There is a medico-legal question as to whether surgery may be based on the results of fine needle biopsy without first obtaining an open biopsy. The answer depends on the experience of the pathologist. Radical surgery has been done based on cytological examination alone. Results indicate that it may be done based on core biopsy paraffin section. Nevertheless, the standard approach is the performance of open biopsy and histological examination by frozen section and/or paraffin section just before surgery.

There are variations in the practice of diagnostic breast biopsy. No single procedure is ideal for all cases. Only after evaluating the patient thoroughly and having considered the advantages and disadvantages of the various methods can a biopsy plan best suited to a particular patient be selected.

One-State Versus Two-Stage Surgery

A one-stage method means a quick frozen section diagnosis of the biopsy specimen followed by immediate surgery. The two-stage method consists of performing only the biopsy at one procedure, awaiting microscopic diagnosis by paraffin section, and then proceeding with surgery at a later date.

The two-stage approach to biopsy and treatment has been recommended by the 1979 National Institute of Health Consensus Conference. It allows time for detailed pathological examination and an opportunity to discuss with the patient subsequent diagnostic and therapeutic procedures.

Delays of 14 to 28 days between biopsy and subsequent surgery have no apparent adverse effect but an increase in infection rates was noted.

Surgery

No treatment for early breast cancer has ever yielded better local control of disease or longterm survival than radical mastectomy and extended radical mastectomy. Despite a recent hypothesis that breast cancer is clearly a systemic disease at the time of clinical presentation, the greatest survivals have been observed with radical mastectomy and modified radical mastectomy and all treatment results are compared to them.

LOCAL EXCISIONS OR PARTIAL MASTECTOMY

Alternatives to mastectomy have become available in recent years for the management of early breast cancer. They consist of a combination of limited surgery, in other words preservation of the breast, and radical radiation therapy. The goal of this approach is to achieve satisfactory local tumor control while preserving the breast.

Treating patients with early breast cancer by local excision and radical therapy was started in Europe and Canada in the 1930s. The results showed longterm survivals but there was a high rate of local recurrence. This was due to the use of irradiation in inadequate doses.

Mistakallio of Helsinki started in the 1930s by treating patients who refused radical mastectomy with local excision and radiation. When he noticed satisfactory results he continued to practice this method. All his patients had T1 and T2 primary tumors, and were given a rad dose of 2500 to 3500 to the breast and regional lymph area. They were followed up for periods of 20 years and compared to a radical mastectomy group. The 20 year survival rates of mastectomy and this group were almost identical – 73% and 78%. The local recurrence rate was higher in the excision group. Since the use of megavoltage therapy, they have observed a significant reduction in their recurrence rate.

Peters from the Princess Margaret hospital in Toronto, Canada reported in 1977 on 203 patients treated between 1939 and 1972 by breast conserving surgery and compared to 600 treated by radical mastectomy. They were followed up for 30 years and the survival without evidence of disease was identical in the two groups.

Data is being accumulated now on the results of treatment by a more modern radiation technique using megavoltage therapy. Noted studies are those of Calle and colleagues at the Foundation Curie in Paris, France, at the Memorial Hospital, and the Marseilles Cancer Institute. They all show that the 10 year disease free survival of patients treated by local excision and radiotherapy is identical to those treated by radical and modified radical mastectomy.

Hellman and associates from the Harvard Joint Center in Boston reported in 1984 their overall experience of treating 357 patients with clinical stage I and II. Most patients received a boost to the primary tumor area by interstitial implantation of irridium Ir-192 delivering an additional dose of 1500-2500 rad. The results of the study showed that the 6 year local tumor control for patients treated by local excision and adequate radiation was 96% for stage I and 90% for stage II breast cancer.

Another significant study emerged from the M.D. Anderson hospital in Houston Texas in 1984. A study of 1000 patients indicated no significant difference in the recurrence rate and survival in patients treated with conservative surgery and radiation, compared with radical or modified mastectomy.

SURGICAL TECHNIQUE IN BREAST PRESERVING PROCEDURES

The surgical procedure should include at least a total excision of the primary tumor with a clear margin. An axillary lymph node dissection is also recommended for the following reasons:

    1.   Histological examination of the nodes will provide infomation on the patient's prognosis.

2. Removal of the nodes will minimize the need for intensive irradiation of the axilla.

3. Patients with positive lymph nodes should receive adjuvant chemotherapy.

Sampling alone might not yield adequate information and when the sample nodes are positive the whole axilla will have to be irradiated anyway.

CONTRAINDICATIONS TO BREAST CONSERVING TREATMENT INCLUDES:

1. Large size of primary lesion in relation to the size of the breast.

2. Location of the primary lesion.
   A lesion under the nipple necessitates removal of the nipple and causes deformity.

3. Multicentricity. Two or more dominant lesions.

4. When the lesion is diffuse and no clear margins can be obtained.

OTHER LIMITATIONS OF RADIOTHERAPY TO CONSIDER IN BREAST PRESERVATION

1. Radiotherapy is ineffective in managing preinvasive breast cancer such as intraductal or lobular carcinoma in situ presumably because they resemble normal breast tissue.

2. Radiotherapy is inferior to adequate surgery for local control of large breast cancers.

3. Radiotherapy requires long and frequent follow-up. After mastectomy local failures occur most frequently in the early years. After radiotherapy, local failures occur at a constant rate over at least 15 years at about 2% a year. Surgical and radiation fibrosis necessitate more frequent physical examinations, mammography, needle aspiration and biopsy.

5. Local excision and radiotherapy offer no advantages over mastectomy in terms of postoperative physical and emotional problems. The only significant difference in numerous factors examined were better body image but more frequent shoulder stiffness in patients with intact breasts.

The only advantage of preserving therapy is the preservation of the breast.

RECURRENCE AND SALVAGE SURGERY – What is done when the lesion recurrs?

Pooling the available information, the 5 year recurrence rate after minimal surgery and irradiation is about 5-6%, the 10 year recurrence rate is 13-14%, and the 15 year recurrence rate is 22%. The local regional recurrence can be effectively treated by salvage treatment. Recurrence in the breast after treatment by limited surgery and radiation behaves biologically different than recurrences which develop after mastectomy. The usual time of recurrence is within two years of mastectomy and it usually signifies poor prognosis. In the case of limited surgery, local recurrence usually occurs at a later date and does not imply a poor prognosis. Most of these patients are suitable for mastectomy with longterm tumor control and survival.

BREAST RECONSTRUCTION

Immediate breast reconstruction is performed only rarely. For patients with small infiltrating cancers and pathologically negative axillary nodes reconstruction may be performed as early as 4-6 months postoperatively. For patients requiring postoperative radiation therapy and/or chemotherapy, in whom the risk of local relapse is much higher, breast reconstruction is ordinarily delayed 6-12 months beyond the completion of all postoperative adjuvant therapy.

THE MANAGEMENT OF CLINICALLY NON-PALPABLE BREAST CANCER

An ever-increasing number of breast cancers are being detected before they can be clinically detected by:

1. Mammography.
2. Histological studies of the tissue surrounding a benign lesion.
3. Studies of tissue removed in random biopsies of the other breast.

4. Studies of the tissues obtained in reduction mammoplasty
    or a prophylactic mastectomy.

Many of these cancers are small and early, and are called:
minimal breast cancer, occult, presymptomatic or preclinical. They
are classified as stage zero or Tis or To or Tlai or Tlbi. It must
be noted that there are cancers larger than 1 cm in size usually
found by mammography that are clinically undetectable mainly in
women with large breasts.

Biopsy of occult lesions may prove difficult. Done under
general anesthesia, the localization is made by obtaining specific
measurements from the radiologist, by tape grid markers, by dye
injection prior to surgery, or by needle localization before
surgery. Treatment of occult cancer is controversial and should be
individualized.

Lobular carcinoma in situ is considered a truly non-invasive
cancer. The variations in the surgical approach range from simple
wide excision to subcutaneous mastectomy, total mastectomy, bilateral mastectomy, and modified radical mastectomy.

We prefer doing bilateral total mastectomy with axillary nodes
sampling, followed by breast reconstruction. This procedure ensures
that no invasive component is left behind.

MANAGEMENT OF SMALL INVASIVE CANCERS

These are treated by breast conserving operation and irradiation or modified radical mastectomy. They have a 90-98% 10 year
survival rate. This excellent prognosis of these early preclinical
cancers emphasizes the importance of early detection. The 10 year
survival of 98% compared to 73% survival of stage I and 43%
survival of stage II.

CONCLUSIONS

When the results of the various primary treatments for
potentially curable breast cancers are compared, variations in
local therapy do not materially affect survival rates. Therefore
the least mutilating surgical procedure may appropriately be
offered to most patients.

The debate over the ideal surgical procedure rests today on differences regarding the handling of the axillary contents.

Is dissection of the entire axillary contents needed? or only sampling? The optimal surgical procedure will be found with clinical trials which depend on the willingness of surgeons and patients to participate in investigative studies to find the ideal operation for breast cancer.

Meanwhile, we do the best we can with the information available to us.

8

Chemotherapy of Breast Cancer

I. Craig Henderson, M.D.

The use of systemic therapy as an adjuvant to mastectomy and/or radiotherapy of local breast cancer has been shown to prolong the time to recurrence for all patients regardless of age and nodal status. In addition, the survival of two groups of patients has been shown to be prolonged by the use of adjuvant therapy. Some patients may be "cured," or have the same life expectancy after adjuvant therapy that they would have had if never diagnosed with breast cancer, but there is at present no evidence that adjuvant therapy cures any patients, and such evidence is not likely to be forthcoming for several decades.

The first adjuvant therapy trials were begun 40 years ago at the Christie Hospital in Manchester, England, when women were randomized to receive either ovarian ablation or no adjuvant therapy. A second generation of trials utilized a short course of perioperative chemotherapy, often given in the operating room and never administered for more than a week or so. However, current standards regarding the use of adjuvant chemotherapy and hormonal therapy are based on trials begun in the early 1970s. In these studies either chemotherapy, tamoxifen, or a combination of these two was given for some months to several years after completion of mastectomy or, less frequently, lumpectomy and radiotherapy. A recent overview or meta-analysis of all such trials completed worldwide (except for the USSR and Japan) demonstrated that the odds of death could be reduced by $14\% \pm 4$ (p = 0.03) when any form of chemotherapy was used. (1) However, when analyzed by age groups, this reduction in mortality was significant only among women under age 50, in whom chemotherapy reduced the odds of death in the first 5 years by $22\% \pm$

6. The effects of a combination of drugs were somewhat longer and reduced the odds of death by 26% ± 7. Regimens employing the combination of cyclophosphamide, methotrexate, and 5-fluorouracil (CMF) were most effective and delayed the death of somewhat more than one third of these women (37% ± 9) beyond 5 years. Adjuvant chemotherapy significantly increased the time to recurrence among women over the age of 50, as well, but the size of the reduction in the recurrence rate was about half that seen in younger women. As a result, very small trends in improved mortality did not approach statistical significance. For women aged 50 and over, the reduction in odds of death from any form of chemotherapy was 4% ± 5, for combination chemotherapy 8% ± 6, and for the use of CMF-type regimens 9% ± 9. At the end of 5 years the difference in survival between the women who received some form of adjuvant chemotherapy was better than that of those randomized to no chemotherapy by 6.9% ± 2 for women under age 50 and 1.2% ± 1.6 for women 50 and over. In these studies patients could have received adjuvant tamoxifen or adjuvant radiotherapy if both the treated and control group received these therapies, and the two groups of patients differed in the administration of adjuvant chemotherapy to only one of the two groups.

An overview of all adjuvant tamoxifen studies provided contrasting results. In these studies, the overall reduction in mortality was 16% ± 3 (p < 0.00001), but the effects on mortality were seen only in women aged 50 and over. In this older group the reduction in the odds of death was 20% ± 3 in contrast to the younger group, where there was a significant reduction in recurrence rate but as yet no reduction in mortality (-1% ± 8). However, among the younger women the trial designs more often involved a comparison of tamoxifen plus chemotherapy with chemotherapy alone; only 1000 women had been randomized worldwide in trials comparing tamoxifen with no adjuvant therapy of any type. Differences in survival at the end of 5 years favor tamoxifen by 5.9% ± 1 in women aged 50 and over but only 0.5% ± 1.9 in those under age 50. There was a trend towards greater effect among those trials in which adjuvant tamoxifen was administered for 2 years or more compared to those in which 6 months or 1 year of tamoxifen was administered, but there has been, as yet, no direct comparison of different durations of tamoxifen therapy.

In contrast to the effects of mastectomy and radiotherapy, the effects of adjuvant chemotherapy and adjuvant tamoxifen are often partial. For example, there is no evidence that a patient who recurs after treatment with mastectomy has a prolongation of her survival as a result of treatment. Either she is cured, or she dies at about the same time she would have died without therapy. Death from breast cancer usually occurs because of metastases disseminated months or years prior to diagnosis, and mastectomy has no effect on these distant tumor deposits. On the other hand, adjuvant systemic therapy may substantially reduce such metastatic deposits without totally eradicating them, and in some patients this delay in the growth of metastatic disease will result in a prolongation of survival without cure of the patient. For this reason it cannot be assumed that a 10% difference in the survival of the treated compared to the untreated patients at the end of 10 years means that only 10% of the patients have benefitted, nor does it mean that this 10% of patients has been "cured." Rather, these differences in survival curves result from a modest and variable effect of therapy on most or all of the treated patients. This is especially true when adjuvant therapy is utilized in node-positive patients, most of whom will eventually die of their disease. Therefore, most of the node-positive patients may potentially benefit from adjuvant therapy. Because of the nature of the effects of adjuvant therapy, trial results might better be expressed as an average prolongation of life. A crude estimate of this figure can be derived from a calculation of the difference in the median survival of the treated patients and the control population in a randomized trial. For example, in the first Milan trial, women were randomized to receive either one year of adjuvant CMF or no adjuvant therapy of any type. At the end of 12 years of follow-up the *difference* in median *disease-free* survival is 43 months for all patients, 109 months for the premenopausal patients, but only 5 months for the postmenopausal women. The difference in median *overall* survival is 36 months, but the median survival of premenopausal women in this study has not yet been reached. Among postmenopausal women entered into the original Milan trial the median survival of postmenopausal women randomized to the *control* arm is 15 months better than that of women randomized to receive adjuvant CMF. This suggests that the difference in medians for premenopausal women, when reached, is likely to be in the range of 3-5 years. These data from the Milan trial suggest that postmenopausal women, who experienced the toxicities of adjuvant CMF therapy for one year, failed to derive either a *net* improvement in disease-free survival or any improvement in overall survival as a result of therapy. In a Scottish trial in which women were randomized to receive either adjuvant tamoxifen or tamoxifenas first systemic therapy at recurrence, the difference in disease-free survival among node-positive patients was 53 months. The difference in median overall survival was 22 months. (2)

Until recently most adjuvant chemotherapy studies enrolled only patients who had histologic nodal involvement. However, the success of adjuvant chemotherapy in younger premenopausal women has led to a series of studies in which adjuvant chemotherapy was tested in node-negative women as well. Three of these studies were recently published (3-5), and in each there was a significant increase in disease-free survival. None of these large studies has yet shown an improvement in overall survival. The results of smaller but somewhat more mature trials in node-negative women provide contradictory results. (2) Two of the smallest show an improvement in overall survival, but others have failed to show even an improvement in disease-free survival. The use of adjuvant chemotherapy in node-negative patients continues to be controversial.

A major problem with the use of adjuvant chemotherapy among node-negative women is the fact that 65% or more of these women will be alive without evidence of recurrence 10 years after diagnosis. Thus, these patients will suffer the toxicities of adjuvant chemotherapy without any potential benefit from therapy since they have ostensibly been cured of their disease with local therapies only. This is particularly important in light of the lack of firm data on the long-term effects of these adjuvant therapies. As yet, the most commonly used adjuvant treatment, CMF, has not been associated with an increased incidence of second tumors. However, L-phenylalanine mustard, used in many of the National Surgical Adjuvant Breast Project (NSABP) trials during the 1970s resulted in an elevenfold increase in acute leukemia. (6) Even adjuvant tamoxifen, which lacks any appreciable acute toxicity, may be associated with an increased incidence in uterine cancer. (7) In one recent report from the Swedish group, adjuvant tamoxifen significantly reduced the incidence of contralateral breast cancers while even more significantly increasing the incidence of uterine cancer.

Because of these late toxicities, there is great emphasis on the search for prognostic factors that will define a distinct group of patients. Such a prognostic factor should ideally be reproducible, and it would be helpful if its biological significance could be defined as well. It may prove valuable to understand whether a particular marker better reflects the metastatic potential or the growth rate of a tumor. Prognostic factors evaluated in the clinic have included the presence or absence of lymph node metastases (a prognostic factor universally accepted as the most reproducible and well-defined), tumor grade, receptor status, labelling indices, flow cytometry, tumor cell ploidy, and oncogenes. Although many studies have shown that patients with a poorly differentiated tumor or one with a high tumor grade have a worse prognosis than patients with well-differentiated tumors, no one has yet shown that these data are reproducible among pathologists. In fact, in one recent study, concordance among two or more pathologists reviewing the same slide was precisely that which might have been anticipated by chance alone. Patients with estrogen or progesterone receptor-negative tumors clearly have a worse survival than those with receptor-positive tumors. However, the predictive value of the receptor is greater among node-positive than node-negative patients. For example, in the recent NSABP trials among node-negative patients, the 4-year disease-free survival among ERP-negative patients was 71%, among ERP-positive patients 77%. (5,8) Although this 6% difference is real, it is clear from these, as well as a variety of other studies, that the 25-35% of node-negative patients who will eventually recur of their disease are not exclusively or primarily receptor-negative patients. The data on other prognostic factors, such as labelling indices, flow cytometry, ploidy, and oncogenes are all at an earlier stage of development. There is an abundance of data demonstrating that patients with high labelling indices have a worse prognosis than those with a lower thymidine labelling index, and studies using flow cytometry seem to correlate well with the larger body of research on labelling indices. However, recent studies utilizing both ploidy and flow cytometry exclusively in in node-negative patients seem to be more useful in defining a group of patients (about 10% of all node-negative patients) who will do extremely well rather than identifying the 25-35% of patients likely to recur. (9) Several oncogenes, especially the HER-2/*neu*, have shown that this is also a prognostic factor, but its full potential in identifying the node-negative patients with the worst prognosis remains to be demonstrated. (10)

In addition to identifying the patients most likely to recur, it would be desirable to identify the patients most likely to benefit from therapy. *A priori* it might be assumed that receptor-negative patients would have a higher growth fraction and thus be more responsive to a cytotoxic agent dependent upon cycling cells. However, the recent adjuvant studies failed to show a greater effect among node-negative patients who are also receptor-negative compared to those who were node-negative and receptor-positive. (4)

At present the use of adjuvant chemotherapy is recommended as routine therapy only among node positive, premenopausal women (or those aged < 50). Adjuvant tamoxifen is recommended for node-positive, receptor-positive patients who are postmenopausal or aged 50 and over. Neither therapy is recommended routinely for node-negative patients. There are multiple potential improvements in adjuvant therapy to be tested in the next generation of studies. Prominent among these are questions related to dose intensity, the use of alternating non-cross-resistance regimens, the administration of fluoropyrimidines followed by leukovorin, the alteration of tumor kinetics with growth factors, the use of antibodies directed at growth factors, or the alteration of cell kinetics with endocrine therapy to increase sensitivity to chemotherapy. Thus far the greatest emphasis has been placed on the development of new strategies for the treatment of patients with the more aggressive forms of breast cancer, but more patients die of the indolent types of breast cancer. For this reason, treatment strategies utilizing therapies such as biological response modifiers and differentiation agents deserves considerable attention as well.

The treatment of metastatic breast cancer has not changed substantially over the past decade in spite of the development of many hypothetical treatment strategies, none of which have been adequately tested as yet. Among these is the use of alternating non-cross-resistant regimens along the lines suggested by Goldie and Coleman, the use of continuous infusion therapies for low growth fraction tumors, the sequential use of methotrexate and 5-fluorouracil to take advantage of the unique pharmacologic interaction of these two drugs, and, most importantly, the use of high-dose therapy.

The currently available therapies have a modest effect on patient survival. (11) This can be illustrated with a number of different approaches. For example, patients randomized to receive combinations of chemotherapy and endocrine therapy have higher response rates than those randomized to receive initial treatment with tamoxifen and chemotherapy only after failure to respond to tamoxifen. However, patients randomized to the combination hormonal/chemotherapy regimens have not been shown to have a better survival in most studies comparing these two treatment strategies. In similar fashion, the use of standard doses of therapy compared to low-dose therapy or the use of chemotherapy for prolonged courses of therapy compared to chemotherapy for 3-month intervals has not resulted in a substantial prolongation of survival in spite of more frequent responses to standard dose therapy or more prolonged duration therapy. (12, 13) Combinations including adjuvant doxorubicin generally induce a higher response than those without doxorubicin, but in all but a few instances this improvement in response has not improved survival. One general exception to this principle is a recent EORTC study in which patients were randomized to receive the classic CMF with cyclophosphamide given orally on days 1-14 and methotrexate intravenously on days 1 and 8. (14) Alternatively, patients received an intravenous CMF in which all drug was given on day 1. In this trial, the response rate to the more traditional or "classical" CMF was 45%, in contrast to the intravenous CMF regimen, to which the response rate was 29% (p = 0.003). The doses of CMF used in the "classic" CMF were higher than in the intravenous CMF, but they more frequently had to be reduced because of toxicity. In this study the use of the classical CMF resulted in a significant prolongation of median survival.

Multiple quality of life studies have shown that regimens associated with a higher response rate are more likely to induce an improved quality of life, even if the more effective therapy is more toxic. This was first shown in a randomized comparison of chemotherapy and endocrine therapy. Chemotherapy resulted in a higher response rate, a marginal improvement in survival, but a highly significant improvement in quality of life despite its toxicity. (15) More recently patients were randomized to receive a standard dose of intravenous CMF compared to half dose CMF. (12) The lower dose CMF was, of course, associated with many fewer side effects, but it also resulted in a significantly lower response rate and a lower quality of life as measured on a Linear Analog Self-Assessment evaluation. A similar relationship between a higher response rate and quality of life was shown in a randomized comparison of continuous chemotherapy and intermittent chemotherapy. (13) Those patients who received chemotherapy continuously until progression of disease had a higher response rate and a better quality of life as measured by the LASA evaluation than those patients whose therapy was discontinued after 3 months in the hope that periods of time off of all toxic therapy would provide better net palliation.

Higher doses of chemotherapy are clearly more effective than lower doses in many (but not all) animal models, and there has been considerable debate and retrospective evaluation of dose in the treatment of breast cancer. (16) The data from such retrospective analyses is contradictory and subject to many methodologic pitfalls. At present there are very few data from randomized controlled trials. In the Canadian trial in which women were randomized to receive standard-dose CMF or low-dose CMF, there was a clear quality-of-life advantage and a marginal survival advantage for standard-dose CMF. However, in a trial from M.D. Anderson, in which women were randomized to standard-dose CAF (cyclophosphamide, doxorubicin, and 5-fluorouracil) or high-dose CAF, no advantage was observed for the group of patients receiving the dose escalation. (17) Only one trial prospectively designed to evaluate dose has been initiated in the adjuvant setting. At the present time no data are available from this study. Based on the available evidence, it is equally plausible that the dose response to chemotherapy in patients with any stage of breast cancer will be either quite shallow or quite steep. Reduction in chemotherapy dose is not recommended, but high-dose therapy, especially the high doses utilized in autologous bone marrow transplant programs, is not recommended outside the context of an ongoing trial.

Chemotherapy for the treatment of metastatic breast cancer should be used primarily for palliation and, therefore, has limited value in the asymptomatic patient. However, when chemotherapy is used, the most effective regimens, not the least toxic, should generally be used, since quality of life studies show that the most effective regimens are associated with the greatest quality of life. In general, the highest response rates are seen with combination chemotherapy programs rather than single agents, with doxorubicin-containing combinations, with treatment programs that exceed 3 months, and possibly with higher dose programs. Although the patients who respond to endocrine therapy are well-defined by both receptor status and clinical characteristics, the patients who benefit most from chemotherapy are identified primarily by a process of exclusion. This includes those patients who are refractory to endocrine therapy, those who have a short disease-free interval and/or negative or low receptor values, and those who have visceral disease.

REFERENCES

1 Early Breast Cancer Trialists Collaborative Group. The Effects
   of Adjuvant Tamoxifen and of Cytotoxic Therapy on Mortality in
   Early Breast Cancer: An Overview of 61 Randomised Trials Among
   28,896 Women. New Engl. J. Med. (1988) 319:1681-1692.

2 Henderson, I. C. Adjuvant Systemic Therapy for Early Breast
   Cancer. Curr. Probl. Cancer (1987) 11:125-207.

3 Ludwig Breast Cancer Study Group. Prolonged Disease-Free Survival after One Course of Perioperative Adjuvant Chemotherapy
   for Node-Negative Breast Cancer. New Engl. J. Med. (1989)
   320:491-496.

4 Mansour, E. G., R. Gray, A. H. Shatila, C. K. Osborne, D. C.
   Tormey, K. W. Gilchrist, M. R. Cooper, G. Falkson. Efficacy of
   Adjuvant Chemotherapy in High-Risk Node-Negative Breast
   Cancer. New Engl. J. Med. (1989) 320:485-490.

5 Fisher, B., C. Redmond, N. Dimitrov, D. Bowman, S. Legault-
   Poisson, D. L. Wickerham, N. Wolmark, E. R. Fisher, R. Mar-
   golese, S, C. Sutherland, A. Glass, R. Foster, R. Caplan. A
   Randomized Clinical Trial Evaluating Sequential Methotrexate
   and Fluorouracil in the Treatment of Patients with Node-
   Negative Breast Cancer Who Have Estrogen-Receptor-Negative
   Tumors. New Engl. J. Med. (1989) 320:473-478.

6 Fisher, B., H. Rockette, E. R. Fisher, D. L. Wickerham, C. Red-
   mond, A. Brown. Leukemia in Breast Cancer Patients Following
   Adjuvant Chemotherapy or Postoperative Radiation: The NSABP
   Experience. J. Clin. Oncol. (1985) 3:1640-1658.

7 Fornander, T., B. Cedermark, A. Mattsson, L. Skoodk, T. Theve,
   J. Askergren, L. E. Rutqvist, U. Glas, C. Silfversward, A.
   Somell, N. Wilking, M. L. Hjalmar. Adjuvant Tamoxifen in Early
   Breast Cancer: Occurrence of New Primary Cancers. Lancet
   (1989) i:117-120.

8 Fisher, B., J. Costantino, C. Redmond, R. Poisson, D. Bowman,
   J. Couture, N. Dimitrov, N. Wolmark, D. L. Wickerham, E. R.
   Fisher, R. Margolese, A. Robidoux, H. Shibata, J. Terz, A. H.
   G. Paterson, M. I. Feldman, W. Farrar, J. Evans, H. L. Lick-
   ley, M. Ketner. A Randomized Clinical Trial Evaluating Tamoxi-
   fen in the Treatment of Patients with Node-Negative Breast
   Cancer Who Have Estrogen-Receptor- Positive Tumors. New Engl.
   J. Med. (1989) 320:479-484.

9 Dressler, L. G., L. C. Seamer, M. A. Owens, G. M. Clark, W. L.
   McGuire. DNA Flow Cytometry and Prognostic Factors in 1331
   Frozen Breast Cancer Specimens. Cancer (1988) 61:420-427.

10   Slamon, D. J., G. M. Clark. Amplification of c-erbB-2 and Aggressive Human Breast Tumors? Response. Science (1988) 240:1796-1798.

11   Henderson, I. C. "Chemotherapy for Advanced Disease". In: Breast Diseases, Harris JR, Hellman S, Henderson IC and Kinne DW.J.B. Lippincott, Co., Phildelphia, 1987.

12   Tannock, I. F., N. F. Boyd, G. DeBoer, C. Erlichman, S. Fine, G. Larocque, C. Mayers, D. Perrault, H. Sutherland. A Randomized Trial of Two Dose Levels of Cyclophosphamide, Methotrexate, and Fluorouracil Chemotherapy for Patients with Metastatic Breast Cancer. J. Clin. Oncol. (1988) 6:1377-1387.

13   Coates, A., V. Gebski, J. F. Bishop, P. N. Jeal, R. L. Woods, R. Snyder, M. H. N. Tattersall, M. Byrne, V. Harvey, G. Gill, J. Simpson, R. Drummond, J. Browne, R. Van Cooten, J. F. Forbes. Improving the Quality of Life During Chemotherapy for Advanced Breast Cancer. New Engl. J. Med. (1987) 317:1490-1495.

14   Englesman, E., R. D. Rubens, J. G. M. Klijn, J. Wildiers, N. Rotmensz, R. Sylvester. Comparison of "Classical CMF" with a Three-weekly Intravenous CMF Schedule in Postmenopausal Patients with Advanced Breast Cancer: An EORTC Study (Trial 10808). Proc. 4th EORTC Breast Cancer Working Conf. (1987) pp. 1-.

15   Baum, M., T. Priestman, R. R. West, E. M. Jones. "A Comparison of Subjective Responses in a Trial Comparing Endocrine with Cytotoxic Treatment in Advanced Carcinoma of the Breast". In: Breast Cancer -- Experimental and Clinical Aspects, Mouridsen HT and Palshof T.Pergamon Press, Oxford, 1980.

16   Henderson, I. C., D. F. Hayes, R. Gelman. Dose Response in the Treatment of Breast Cancer: A Critical Review. J. Clin. Oncol. (1988) 6:1501-1515.

17   Hortobagyi, G. N., A. U. Buzdar, G. P. Bodey, S. Kau, V. Rodriguez, S. S. Legha, H. Yap, G. R. Blumenschein. High-Dose Induction Chemotherapy of Metastatic Breast Cancer in Protected Environment: A Prospective Randomized Study. J. Clin. Oncol. (1987) 5:178-184.

9

MECHANISMS OF ANTICANCER DRUG RESISTANCE

Adrian L. Harris, ICRF Clinical Oncology Unit, Churchill Hospital, Headington, Oxford, OX3 7LJ, England

Introduction

Chemotherapy is essential in the cure of a minority of adult tumours and the majority of childhood tumours. Prolongation of survival by chemotherapy has been proven for breast carcinoma, oat cell lung carcinoma and ovarian carcinoma. However, in many solid tumours such as colo-rectal carcinoma, melanoma and gliomas, response to chemotherapy occurs in less than 20% of cases. Also, even Hodgkins disease and testicular teratoma may relapse and become drug resistant. Thus resistance to chemotherapy is a major problem either de novo or acquired after therapy. Understanding the mechanisms may be helpful for selecting patients for therapy and for new drug development.

Mechanisms of drug resistance can be considered to operate from the point of drug administration to the final achievement of cytocidal drug concentrations at the target site. This review will concentrate particularly on cellular biochemical mechanisms, rather than physiological, pharmacokinetic or drug access and transport mechanisms [1].

There are four major groups of cellular mechanisms:

1)   Multidrug resistance - pleiotropic drug resistance

2)   Metabolic inactivation of nucleophiles
        a) glutathione transferases
        b) glutathione peroxidase
        c) metallothionein
        d) free radical metabolising enzymes

3)   Changes in target expression
        a) gene amplification
        b) point mutations
        c) down regulation of genes

4)   DNA repair

Many of these mechanisms were initially discovered by investigating mammalian cell lines made resistant to drugs in vitro. However, in several cases, using the probes available from these studies, or following up in vitro observations, has shown the relevance of the observations to clinical biopsies and human drug resistance.

1. Multidrug Resistance

This has been studied by making mammalian cells resistant to cytotoxic drugs in vitro, by continued incremental exposure. For resistance induced by some drugs, cells are resistant not only to the drug to which they were exposed, but also to a wide range of drugs with different structures and biochemical mechanisms of action. The drugs involved include adriamycin, VP16, mitoxantrone, vincristine, vinblastine, actinomycin D, melphalan and mitomycin C, all commonly used in human cancer therapy. The mechanism is a membrane pump that is energy dependent and can extrude the anticancer drugs rapidly [2].

In the tumour cell lines resistant to cytotoxic drugs in vitro, it was possible to produce gene amplification of genes critical for multidrug resistance. These amplified genes were cloned and it was shown that transfection of the gene into another cell could produce multidrug resistance. This was the human multidrug resistance gene (mdr 1).

The gene product is the P-glycoprotein. The role of the protein in normal tissues is unclear, but it is located at the luminal surface of the colon and biliary tract epithelium, the luminal surface of the proximal renal tubules and in the adrenal cortex. It may therefore have an excretory and protective function against environmental toxins.

It has been shown to be highly expressed in the majority of tumours arising from organs that normally express P-glycoprotein e.g. colon tumours, hypernephroma, pancreatic and adrenal carcinoma. It is not commonly expressed in chemosensitive haemopoeitic tumours de novo, but is expressed on relapse. It has also been demonstrated to increase during development of drug resistant ovarian carcinoma. Thus it is an important mechanism of de novo and acquired drug resistance.

The structure of P-glycoprotein is very similar to previously cloned E coli genes involved in excretion of haemolysin and the transport of aminoacids. This homology is maintained in function, so that P-glycoprotein transports a wide range of cytotoxic drugs. Recently it has been shown that point mutations in the internal domain can confer specifically much higher resistance to one drug than another [3]. Thus the pattern of cross resistance may be different depending on the initial drugs used. Although this mechanism explains much about drug resistance and sensitivity, it does not appear to be related to sensitivity to crosslinking agents, cisplatinum, bleomycin, antimetabolites or X-rays. Hence there remain many other mechanisms that could be modulated and provide the basis for selective toxicity.

2 Metabolic Inactivation of Nucleophiles

a) Glutathione transferases

The glutathione transferases (GSTs) are multi-functional proteins that protect cells agains carcinogens and many other toxins. The GST conjugate reduced glutathione (GSH) with a wide variety of xenobiotics and this facilitates the elimination of the latter, since the resulting metabolites are more water soluble. GSTs can also bind some lipophilic compounds and either prevent them interacting with DNA or act as carrier proteins (ligands) assisting hepatic removal and biliary excretion of foreign compounds [4].

There are four major classes of human GST, a microsomal GST and three cytosolic groups - acidic, neutral and basic. The cytosolic enzymes exist as homo or heterodimers. The acidic transferases are known as Yf (or π), the neutral as Yb_1, Yb_2, Yn (or μ) and the basic as Ya, Yc, Yk (or a). Ya type subunits consist of two types B_1 and B_2 which can exist as B_1B_1, B_1B_2 or B_2B_2.

Each major class or glutathione transferases has a wide range of substrates, which overlaps with the other classes. However there are preferred substrates within each class which are used as an enzymatic method to discriminate between the transferases.

Because they interact with such a wide range of nucleophiles, it may be expected that elevation of GSTs may be a mechanism of cytotoxic drug resistance. Melphalan-glutathione adducts can be formed much more rapidly in the presence of human liver cytosolic GSTs [5]. Evidence for a role of GSTs in drug resistance comes from two sources; assay of GSTs in parent sensitive and derived resistant cell lines, and by modulating glutathione levels.

The drug buthionine-(SR)-sulfoximine (BSO) inhibits g glutamyl cysteine synthetase, a key enzyme in glutathione biosynthesis [6]. Levels of depletion down to about 10% of normal can be achieved without much toxicity. If this drug markedly potentiates cytotoxicity of an anticancer drug, this is circumstantial evidence for a role of glutathione in protection against that particular agent. Drugs for which this has been reported include the mustards such as melphalan, chlorambucil and nitrogen mustard and also cyclophosphamide, adriamycin and cisplatinum.

We and others have developed cell lines resistant to alkylating agents and demonstrated elevation of glutathione transferases. We used chlorambucil which is active in breast cancer as well as chronic lymphoid leukaemia. The particular types of GST included increased acidic GST and also increased expression of a basic GST, Yc. In addition there were increases in activity of enzymes involved in glutathione synthesis and salvage and a rise in glutathione levels [7].

Thus the glutathione/GSTs system can produce broad spectrum drug resistance, and also radiation resistance. However modification of glutathione levels by BSO is under phase 1 study currently, and may overcome this mechanism in some cases.

b)   Glutathione peroxidase

Glutathione peroxidase activity is a feature of the glutatione transferases and another enzyme - selenium dependent glutathione peroxidase. Although both can act on organic peroxides, only the latter acts on hydrogen peroxide. In breast cancer cell lines made resistant to adriamycin, there was a marked increase in the selenium dependent form [8]. There was also increased expression of the multidrug resistance gene, showing that there are often multiple mechanisms of resistance in resistant cells.

c)   Metallothionein

Metallothioneins are low molecular weight proteins (6000-7000) with an extremely high sulphur and metal content, up to 20% of their weight [9]. They bind metals via their cysteine residues, and the order of affinity is cadmium>lead>zinc. There are two major groups of metallothionein MT-1 and MT-2, but as many as ten iso-MT genes are expressed in humans. They function in heavy metal homeostasis and detoxification. The abundant sulphydryl groups (20 per molecule) can interact with toxins and scavenge oxygen free radicals. Human carcinoma cells transfected with the human metallothionein II_A gene became resistant to cisplatinum, melphalan chlorambucil and to a small extent adriamycin [10]. Metallothionein expression can be induced by the H*ras* oncogene and this is a potential reason for drug resistance in some human cancers.

d)   Free radical metabolising enzymes

Many cytotoxic drugs generate free radicals as part of their mechanisms of action eg adriamycin, bleomycin, mytomycin C, VP16. There are many other enzymes besides the glutathione peroxidases and transferases involved in the detoxification of free radicals. Examples include superoxide dismutase and catalase [11].

3)   Changes in target expression

a)   Gene amplification

In the past ten years gene amplification has been found to be a mechanism for experimental drug resistance in cultured mammalian cells.   The extra copies of DNA result in cytologically enlarged regions on chromosomes (homogenously staining regions) or reside on extrachromosomal self-replicating elements (double minutes) [12].

In most cases the gene is an enzyme critical for a biochemichal pathway involved in DNA synthesis and increased gene dosage results in increased mRNA and production of the enzyme.   There is thus a large excess of enzyme that cannot be inhibited sufficiently by clinically achievable drug concentrations.   The classical example is dihydrofolate reductase (DHFR), the target for methotrexate.   Gene amplification has been demonstrated for DHFR in vivo in patients whose tumours are resistant to methotrexate, but the general importance of this mechanism in vivo is poorly defined in human cancer.   However far greater degrees of resistance can be achieved by amplification than any other mechanism.

Apart from the specific changes in target genes, multidrug resistance genes and glutathione transferases may also be amplified, conferring broad spectrum resistance as discussed earlier.

b) Point mutations

Another mechanism that can greatly change the affinity of a drug for its target is mutation in the region of the gene coding for the drug-binding domain of the enzyme.

Abnormal thymidylate synthetase has been reported in resistance to 5FUdR, and also a mutated topoisomerase I resistant to camptothecin (a topoisomerase inhibitor) [13].

The multidrug resistance gene can also be mutated such that its product has much greater affinity for one class of drug, and hence produces much greater resistance to that drug than others.

c) Down regulation of genes - topoisomerase II

The loss of specific transporters for folates has been related to resistance to antimetabolites such as methotrexate.   Similarly the increased expression of the purine salvage pathway enzyme hypoxynthine guanine phosphoribosyl transferase is associated with resistance to thiopurines (6MP, 6TG).   The mechanism regulating these changes include deletion of the genes, or methylation of the genes.

A key enzyme target for a wide range of drugs - topoisomerase II - is commonly down regulated in multidrug resistant cells, in addition to the increase in P-glycoprotein and glutathione transferase expression. The mechanisms regulating topoisomerase II are currently unknown.

Topoisomerase II is composed of homologous dimers of approximately 170 Kd each [14]. It can transiently break and reseal both strands of double stranded DNA, and allow passage of another double stranded DNA through the breaks.

The topo II is covalently bound to the 5' end of the breaks during the breakage-revision cycle. This is known as a "cleavable complex" and results in a protein associated DNA break. There are several different enzymatic activities of topo II, including the ability to unknot DNA, to decatenate circular interlocked DNA and reduction of supercoiling. Topo II also appears to act as a structural protein, anchoring DNA to the nuclear scaffold. Topo II therefore has roles in DNA transcription (releasing local increases in supercoiling) replication, chromosome segregation, sister chromatid exchange and recombination.

The drugs that are known to interact with topoisomerase II and trap in in its DNA-bound form include adriamycin, daunorubicin, VP16, VM26, mitoxantrone, ellipticine, m-AMSA and actomycin D. It appears that this trapped cleavable complex may interfere with DNA replication by obstructing movement of a replication complex along DNA. Since the number of protein associated breaks depends on the amount of topoisomerase II (each break requiring two molecules of topo II) then the more topo II, the more breaks and the greater obstruction to DNA synthesis. This has been shown to be the case in mutant cell lines expressing different amounts of topo II [15], and explains how a reduction in topo II could be a major mechanism of resistance to many clincally used drugs.

4)   DNA Repair

The importance of basal DNA repair mechanisms in carcinogenesis and cytotoxicity is suggested by the human repair deficiency diseases. Cell lines from patients with ataxia telangiectasia are hypersensitive to topoisomerase II inhibitors [16]. Xeroderma pigmentosum cells are hypersensitive to UV and cisplatinum. Fanconi's anaemia cells are hypersensitive to DNA cross linking agents. These patients are at increased risk of a variety of haemopoietic neoplasms or solid tumours.

There are over 100 genes in E-coli involved in DNA repair, with several different pathways for different types of lesion. There is also considerable redundancy and overlap. The situation is likely to be even more complex in human cells. Apart from the familial repair defects, there are over 40 mammalian repair mutants reported [17]. Thus 'DNA repair' covers a wide range of enzyme activities including repair of DNA single strand breaks, double strand breaks, recombination, repair of mismatched bases, crosslinks, monoadducts and alkylated bases. For each DNA-binding drug there are likely to be several repair enzymes involved and different enzymes for different drugs. However in a few cases there do seem to be particular repair enzymes critical to protection against one class of drugs.

a) O^6alkyl guanine alkyltransferase

Nitrosureas such as BCNU, CCNU alkylate DNA at a particular site on guanine - the O^6 atom. Crosslinks are formed via intramolecular recombination from this site to the C_3 position and then to an adjacent guanine residue.

A specific repair enzyme recognises the O^6 lesions and dealkylates guanine residues, covalently attaching the alkyl group to a cysteine residue in the protein [18]. This inactivates the protein irreversibly - hence the enzymes is acting as a suicide repair protein. Human tissues have much higher levels of this enzyme than mouse or rat tissues. Although nitrosoureas are amongst the most active drugs ever detected on murine tumour screens, they are of relatively poor activity in human cancer. The main reason is probably the marrow suppression (since marrow has very low levels of the repair enzyme) and high expression of the enzyme in tumours. However, there are occasional responses to nitrosureas, and DTIC also alkylates guanine in the O^6 position [19]. Thus assay of this enzyme in tumours allow selection of patients with low levels.

b) Cisplatinum repair

Cisplatinum produces mainly intrastrand DNA crosslinks and in cell lines there is good evidence that rapid repair is one mechanism related to drug resistance [20].

In patients treated with cisplatinum, the DNA crosslinks can be measured in peripheral leucocytes by immunoassay. In patients responding to cisplatinum, more crosslinks were detected in their peripheral leucocytes [21]. This was not due to differences in cisplatinum pharmacokinetics. The most reasonable explanation is that there are genetic variations in repair of DNA damage, and that the differences are also manifest in tumours. Thus patients whose normal tissues repair cisplatinum adducts slowly, ie have high levels of adducts in their leucocytes, also have tumours with poor repair. These are the tumours that are therefore more sensitive to chemotherapy.

If these results are confirmed by direct measurements in tumours, it would suggest that inhibiting DNA repair may potentiate chemotherapy in drug resistant tumours.

Conclusions

There are multiple mechanisms for resistance to chemotherapy. There may be several mechanisms for one drug, or one mechanism may give resistance to several drugs. More than one mechanism may be expressed simultaneously.

However, in each case, understanding the mechanism provides the basis for clinical interventions to overcome drug resistance (eg verapamil for multidrug resistance) or provides a basis for new drug development (eg drugs activated by glutathione transferases, or topo II inhibitors not transported by P-glycoprotein).

Patients will need to be selected for such studies by assays of the relevant resistance mechanism in tumour biopsies, and randomised comparisons of the modulation plus chemotherapy versus chemotherapy alone need to be performed.

References

1. Harris, A. L. Advanced Medicine (Ed. Ferguson, A.) Pitman Publishing Ltd., London, 1984, pp. 313-362.

2. Bradley, G., Juranka, P. F. and Ling, V. Biochim. & Biophys. Acta. 948:87-128, 1988.

3. Choi, K., Chen, C., Kriegler, M. and Roninson, I.B. Cell, 53: 519-529, 1988.

4. Mannervik, B. (Ed. Meister, A.), Advances in Enzymology, 57: 357-417, 1985.

5. Dulik, D. M., Fenselav, C. and Hilton, J. Biochem. Pharmacol. 35:3405-3409, 1986.

6. Skapek, S. X., Colvin, O. M., Griffith, O. W., Elion, G. B., Bigner, D. D. and Friedman, H. S. Cancer Res., 48:2764-2767, 1988.

7. Lewis, A. D., Hickson, I. D., Robson, C. N., Harris, A. L., Hayes, J. D., Griffiths, S. A., Manson, M. M., Hall, A. E., Moss, J. E., Wolf, C. R., Proc. Natl. Acad. Sci. USA, 85:8511-8515, 1988.

8. Kagi, J. H. R. and Schaffer, A. Biochem. 27:28510-8515, 1988.

9. Kelley, S. L., Basu, A., Teicher, B. A., Hacker, M. P., Hamer, D. H. and Lazo, J. S. Science 241:1813-1815, 1988.

10. Kramer, R. A., Zakher, J. and Kim, G.   Science 241: 694-697, 1988.

11. Hall, A. H. Jr. Eanes, E. Z., Waymack, P. P. Jr. and Patterson, R. M., Mutat. Res. 198:166-168, 1988.

12. Stark, G. R., Cancer Surveys 5:1-23, 1986.

13. Kjeldsen, E., Bonven, B. J., Andoh, T., Ishii, K., Okada, K., Bolund, L. and Westergaard, O.   J. Biol. Chem. 263:3912-3916, 1988.

14. Drlica, K. and Franco, R. J.   Biochem. 27:2253-2259, 1988.

15. Davies, S. M., Robson, C. N., Davies, S. L. and Hickson, I. D. J. Biol. Chem. 263:17724-17729, 1988.

16. Davies, S. M., Harris, A. L. and Hickson, I. D. Nucl. Acid. Res. (in press)

17. Hickson, I. D. and Harris, A. L. TIGS 4:101-106, 1988.

18. Harris, A. L., Karran, P. and Lindahl, T.   Cancer Res. 43: 3247-3252, 1983.

19. Lunn, J. M. and Harris, A. L. Br. J. Cancer 57:54-58

20. Eastman, A. and Schulte, N. Biochem. 27:4730-4734, 1988.

21. Reed, E., Ozols, R. F., Tarone, R., Yuspa, S. H. and Poirier, M. Proc. Natl. Acad. Sci. USA 84:5024-5028, 1987.

10

MULTIDRUG-RESISTANCE IN HUMAN CANCER

M.M. GOTTESMAN, L.J. GOLDSTEIN, H. GALSKI AND I. PASTAN

Laboratory of Molecular Biology, National Cancer Institute,
National Institutes of Health, Bethesda, Maryland, U.S.A. 20892

INTRODUCTION

Primary treatment of early stage breast cancer is by surgery
and radiation therapy. Cure is frequently achieved if the cancer
has not spread. Recent studies suggest that the addition of
adjuvant chemotherapy can increase the long-term survival of
patients with breast cancer, presumably by killing cancer cells
beyond the operative field, and that use of chemotherapy after
recurrence of breast cancer can provide significant palliation.
However, all too often breast cancer recurs after chemotherapy and
appears to be resistant to further chemotherapeutic maneuvers.
Thus, the problem of acquired drug-resistance in breast cancer is a
major one, and efforts to improve chemotherapy of breast cancer
must be based on knowledge of the mechanism or mechanisms by which
breast cancer cells become resistant to chemotherapy.

One major way in which cultured cancer cells, including human
breast cancer cells, become resistant to certain kinds of
chemotherapy involves the expression of the multidrug-resistance,
or MDR1 gene (reviewed in 1 and 2). This gene has been cloned from
several different human and rodent cell lines based on the fact
that the MDR1 gene frequently becomes amplified and its mRNA is
overexpressed in cells selected for resistance to drugs such as
doxorubicin (Adriamycin), daunomycin, vincristine, vinblastine, and
actinomycin D. Some of these drugs, especially doxorubicin and the
Vinca alkaloids, are agents used in the treatment of breast cancer.

The human MDR1 gene is transcribed into a 4.5 kb mRNA which
encodes a 1280 amino acid protein (3). The multidrug-resistance

protein is a 170,000 dalton molecular weight plasma membrane protein, also called P-glycoprotein (2). Cells which express this protein are resistant to drugs because they fail to accumulate these drugs in their cytoplasm. Although the drugs are rapidly taken up by the cells, they are quickly pumped out by an energy-dependent multidrug transport system.

Several lines of evidence indicate that P-glycoprotein is the multidrug transporter: (1) Using specific antisera to P-glycoprotein, it has been localized to the plasma membrane of resistant cells, consistent with its function as a pump (4); (2) Photoactivatable, radiolabeled analogs of drugs which are transported by the multidrug transport system are affinity labels of P-glycoprotein (5, 6); (3) An ATP analog binds specifically to P-glycoprotein (7); (4) Vesicles containing P-glycoprotein formed from multidrug-resistant cells are capable of transporting drugs in an ATP-dependent manner (8); (5) Several drugs which are known to reverse the multidrug-resistance phenotype, including verapamil and quinidine, inhibit the affinity-labeling of P-glycoprotein (5) and also block transport into P-glycoprotein-containing vesicles (8); and (6) When a cDNA encoding P-glycoprotein is cloned into a eukaryotic expression vector and introduced into drug-sensitive cells, they become drug-resistant (9, 10). This experiment proves that overexpression of P-glycoprotein is by itself sufficient to render cells multidrug-resistant, presumably because P-glycoprotein is the multidrug transporter.

Having established that expression of the MDR1 gene in tissue culture cells results in a multidrug-resistant phenotype, it was important to determine whether expression of this gene occurs in normal human tissues and cancers, and whether it plays a role in clinical drug-resistance. Using specific cDNA probes for MDR1 RNA and specific antisera for P-glycoprotein, MDR1 expression was found in epithelial tissues of several normal organs including kidney, liver, colon, adrenal and small intestine, and also in brain and testis capillary endothelial cells (11-13). The P-glycoprotein was localized in these cells in a polarized fashion, consistent with a possible role as a transporter in these tissues. One possibility is that it functions as a protection against toxic, natural products in our diet which are synthesized by plants and micro-organisms. Since the transporter shows very little specificity, another possibility is that it transports a variety of endogenous metabolites, and that these metabolites might differ in different tissues.

A minimum requirement to prove a role of P-glycoprotein in clinical drug-resistance is the demonstration that the MDR1 gene is expressed in human cancer. This paper summarizes the results of the analysis of over 400 human cancers and unselected human cancer cell lines for the presence of MDR1 RNA. As will become apparent, expression of the MDR1 gene is widespread in many human cancers. Expression occurs in breast cancer as well, and preliminary data suggest that the incidence of this expression is increased in tumors refractory to chemotherapy.

RESULTS AND DISCUSSION

Several assays are available for the detection of MDR1 RNA or P-glycoprotein. Immunological detection of P-glycoprotein appeared to be less sensitive than detection of RNA using cDNA probes. Therefore, we chose to measure MDR1 RNA, rather than protein in these studies. RNA can be measured by in situ analysis (14), which gives information about the distribution of MDR1 RNA in individual cells, but is somewhat less sensitive (because of non-specific background) than an assay which measures total MDR1 RNA in a population of cells. In practice, we prepare RNA from frozen tumor specimens, and make multiple dilutions of this RNA on a slot blot apparatus. The amount of RNA is estimated by detection of ribosomal RNA bands on agarose gels, and equal loading of RNA is confirmed on the slot blots by comparison of the signal generated using a γ-actin probe. Use of a radioactive probe for the human MDR1 gene produces a signal proportional to the amount of RNA on the blot. This signal intensity can be compared to that of a standard drug sensitive cell line (KB-3-1) or a cell line (KB-8-5) which is 3-6-fold resistant to various drugs and expresses approximately 30-fold as much RNA as the standard drug sensitive line. The KB-8-5 RNA level is arbitrarily given a value of 30 units of MDR1 RNA. Details of this assay have been described (15). This assay is sensitive, reproducible, and specific for MDR1 RNA, as confirmed with different MDR1 probes and RNAse protection assays (15).

We have used the MDR1 slot blot assay to measure MDR1 RNA levels in over 400 human cancers (15). Based on these assay results, it is possible to divide these human cancers into five groups:

(1) Tumors which express elevated levels of MDR1 RNA in at least 50% of tested samples. This group includes cancers derived from tissues which normally express MDR1 RNA such as colon carcinoma, renal cell carcinoma, hepatoma, adrenocortical cancer, pheochromocytomas, and pancreatic islet cell tumors. In addition, frequent high level expression of MDR1 RNA is found in carcinoid tumors, non-small cell lung cancer with neuroendocrine properties (NSCLC-NE), and chronic myelogenous leukemia in blast crisis (levels in the chronic phase are low). All of these tumors are known to be intrinsically resistant to chemotherapy with Adriamycin or Vinca alkaloids, with the possible exception of the NSCLC-NE, which are somewhat responsive to chemotherapy compared to NSCLC. Since expression of MDR1 RNA is usually associated with the expression of the multidrug transporter, which confers multidrug-resistance in cells in which it is expressed, we interpret these results to mean that at least some of the intrinsic resistance of these cancers is due to expression of the MDR1 gene.

(2) Cancers with occasionally high level expression of the MDR1 gene. Untreated non-Hodgkin's lymphoma and acute adult lymphocytic and non-lymphocytic leukemias express MDR1 RNA in 10-20% of cases, and childhood neuroblastoma was positive in 50% of cases. These results are of special interest since all of these cancers are responsive to chemotherapy, but a minority of the patients have refractory disease which does not respond to chemotherapy. It will be of interest to determine whether the

level of MDR1 RNA expression is a predictor of the response to
chemotherapy in this group.

(3) Cancers in which MDR1 RNA levels are generally low, but
1/3 or fewer show low, but detectable MDR1 RNA signals. These
tumors include breast cancer, non-small cell lung cancer and
bladder cancer. It is difficult to know whether the low positive
signal represents heterogeneity of the cell population with only a
small percentage of cells being breast cancer cells, heterogeneity
of the tumor population, with a small percent of cells having a lot
of MDR1 RNA, or whether most of the breast cancer cells have a low
signal. The correct interpretation of these results will have
important clinical implications. If a low percentage of cells
express high levels of MDR1 RNA, then chemotherapy will select out
this population quickly. Such a result would explain the rapid
emergence of drug-resistant cells in a population, and might
account for only transient responses to chemotherapy in some of
these tumors.

(4) Cancers in which MDR1 RNA levels are usually low. Many
of these cancers are known to be at least partially drug-sensitive
including small cell lung cancer, CML in chronic phase, ovarian
cancer, thymoma, thyroid cancer, Wilm's tumor, sarcoma, and
prostate cancer. Some of the tumors are relatively multidrug-
resistant including melanoma, mesothelioma, esophageal and gastric
carcinoma, and head and neck cancer. This latter result suggests
that other mechanisms must exist to account for the clinical
multidrug-resistance of many tumors.

(5) Cancers which show increased MDR1 RNA levels after
chemotherapy. In some ways this is the most interesting group and
the one in which it may be possible to improve response to chemotherapy. This group includes treated non-Hodgkin's lymphoma, acute
childhood and adult lymphocytic leukemia, acute non-lymphocytic
leukemia of adults, pheochromocytoma, neuroblastoma, ovarian cancer
and breast cancer.

Although our sample population with treated breast cancer is
small (only 3 treated patients, 2 of whom showed elevated MDR1 RNA
levels), the incidence of elevated MDR1 RNA in untreated breast

cancer is low (only 9 of 57 patients). We are currently attempting to study more samples from breast cancer patients relapsing after therapy to see if we can confirm that treatment increases the frequency of MDR1 RNA expression. If this proves to be a reproducible phenomenon, then this evidence would suggest that expression of the MDR1 gene plays an important role in the development of clinical drug resistance in breast cancer.

CONCLUSIONS AND FUTURE PROSPECTS

We have found that expression of the MDR1 gene occurs widely in human cancer. The weight of experimental evidence suggests that the presence of MDR1 RNA signals the presence of the multidrug-resistance phenotype. Thus, it should be possible to use a positive MDR1 RNA assay to guide more rational chemotherapy.

Studies in cultured cell systems have identified several compounds which are able to reverse the multidrug-resistance phenotype, including drugs such as verapamil, quinidine, reserpine, cyclosporin, phenothiazines, and many other natural products. Most of these compounds appear to reverse resistance by inhibiting the pump activity of the multidrug-transporter, probably as competitive inhibitors (1). Non-toxic analogs of these and other reversing agents are under development, and clinical trials of agents such as verapamil and quinidine are in progress. These studies will tell us whether it is feasible to reverse multidrug resistance in animal models and human cancer, without undue host toxicity. If these reversing agents are found to be safe and effective, it may be possible to use them to circumvent clinical drug-resistance of intrinsically resistant tumors, or overcome the drug-resistance of tumors which acquire resistance on the basis of MDR1 RNA expression.

REFERENCES
1. Gottesman, M.M. and Pastan, I. J. Biol. Chem. 263: 12163-12166, 1988.
2. Bradley, G., Juranka, P.F., and Ling, V. Biochim. Biophys. Acta. 948: 87-128, 1988.

3. Chen, C.-j., Chin, J.E., Ueda, K., Clark, D., Pastan, I., Gottesman, M.M., and Roninson, I.B. Cell 47: 381-389, 1986.

4. Willingham, M.C., Richert, N.D., Cornwell, M.M., Tsuruo, T., Hamada, H.,Gottesman, M.M. and Pastan, I. J. Histochem. Cytochem. 35: 1451-1456, 1987.

5. Cornwell, M.M., Safa, A.R., Felsted, R.L., Gottesman, M.M. and Pastan, I. Proc. Natl. Acad. Sci. USA. 83: 3847-3850, 1986.

6. Safa, A.R., Glover, C.J., Sewell, J.L., Meyers, M.B., Biedler, J.L. and Felsted, R.L. J. Biol. Chem. 262: 7884-7888, 1987.

7. Cornwell, M.M., Tsuruo, T., Gottesman, M.M. and Pastan, I. The FASEB J. 1: 51-54, 1987.

8. Horio, M., Gottesman, M.M. and Pastan, I. Proc. Natl. Acad. Sci. USA. 85: 3580-3584, 1988.

9. Gros, P., Ben-Neriah, Y., Croop, J. and Housman, D.E. Nature 323: 28-731, 1986.

10. Ueda, K., Cardarelli, C., Gottesman, M.M. and Pastan, I. Proc. Natl. Acad. Sci. USA 84: 3004-3008, 1987.

11. Fojo, A.T., Ueda, K., Slamon, D.J., Poplack, D.G., Gottesman, M.M. and Pastan, I. Proc. Natl. Acad. Sci. USA. 84: 265-269, 1987.

12. Thiebaut, F., Tsuruo, T., Hamada, H., Gottesman, M.M., Pastan, I. and Willingham, M.C. Proc. Natl. Acad. Sci. USA 84: 7735-7738, 1987.

13. Thiebaut, F., Tsuruo, T., Hamada, H., Gottesman, M.M., Pastan, I. and Willingham, M.C. J. Histochem. Cytochem. 37: 159-164, 1989.

14. Shen, D.-W., Pastan, I. and Gottesman, M.M. Canc. Res. 48: 4334-4339, 1988.

15. Goldstein, L.J., Galski, H., Fojo, A., Willingham, M.C., Lai, S.-L., Gazdar, A., Pirker, R., Green, A., Crist, W., Brodeur, G.M., Lieber, M., Cossman, J., Gottesman, M.M. and Pastan, I. J. Natl. Canc. Inst. 81: 116-124, 1989.

11

HIGH-DOSE CHEMOTHERAPY INTENSIFICATION WITH BONE MARROW SUPPORT FOR HORMONE RECEPTOR NEGATIVE OR HORMONAL REFRACTORY RELAPSING BREAST CANCER.

FRANK R. DUNPHY II, GARY SPITZER, AMAN U. BUZDAR, GABRIEL N. HORTOBAGYI, FRANKIE HOLMES, LEONARD J. HORWITZ, JONATHAN C. YAU, JORGE A. SPINOLO, SUNDAR JAGANNATH and KAREL A. DICKE

University of Texas M.D. Anderson Cancer Center, Houston, TX, USA

HISTORICAL BACKGROUND

From 1975 through 1977 high-dose therapy (HDT) with autologous bone marrow transplant (ABMT) as a strategy to improve survival and response rates in non-hematologic malignancies was first initiated in 13 small cell lung carcinoma (SCLC) patients. The drugs which we initially selected were Cyclophosphamide and Etoposide (VP-16) at doses 4.5 g/m^2 and 750 mg/m^2 respectively, followed by bone marrow infusion on day 5 post HDT. SCLC was selected because of its known chemosensitivity to a number of myelotoxic agents, an impressive complete response rate to conventional chemotherapy in patients with limited disease, yet the disappointingly low percentage of cures (1). Cyclophosphamide and VP-16 were chosen as the initial core drugs in our studies not only because of their known clinical activity but also because of their predominant marrow toxicity. The extramedullary toxicity of these two drugs is modest and rapidly reversible below certain critical levels (Cyclophosphamide below 6 G/m^2 and VP-16 below 1500 mg/m^2). We wished to initially construct our HDT in a sequential manner that would not have as its dose-limiting toxicity extramedullary manifestations but instead be limited by marrow suppression. The emphasis and concerns over designing an approach of HDT that would not have limiting extramedullary toxicities such as hepatic (veno-occlusive disease), pulmonary (interstitial pneumonitis), vascular (thrombotic thrombocytopenia purpuria), was based on our poor insight into the physiology of the repair of these vital structures and therefore our limited knowledge of how to approach the modification of toxicity to such organs. On the contrary, we felt the issue of dose limiting myelosuppression could potentially be markedly modified because of the approaching era of recombinant growth factors and understanding methods of how to expand hematopoietic stem cells and progenitor cells *in vivo* and *in vitro*.

From the initiation of our studies in SCLC we made the commitment to develop a double HDT approach as a method to deliver more aggressive therapy without crossing into the area of serious extramedullary toxicity. With these drugs and this strategy we felt encouraged that indeed we were able to treat a patient population of heavy smokers with advanced age who had significant lung disease from long-term tobacco use. We had no mortality in this initial group and morbidity was very acceptable limited to infectious complications (1).

From 1978 until 1985 an additional 32 SCLC patients were treated with this approach. Drug doses were modestly escalated over the early study and attempts at introducing adriamycin and methotrexate were made. Again the therapy was remarkably well tolerated; there was no therapy related mortality; and the introduction of the additional drugs did not increase the frequency of mucositis or documented infectious episodes. There were six observed long-term disease-free survivors. Examining the clinical features of these six patients we find all six received two cycles of HDT and that five of these were given HDT while in complete remission followed by local radiation consolidation to prior sites of bulky disease. These results strengthened our hypothesis that at the doses used the subset of patients with responsive disease and minimal tumor burden at the time of HDT are the patients most likely to benefit from this approach. Additionally we felt these six long-term survivors supported the principle of delivering two cycles of HDT and of local consolidation with radiotherapy (2).

After 1985 cisplatinum at doses initially of 120 mg/m² in each cycle was introduced to the cyclophosphamide and VP-16 drug combination because of its known synergism with both drugs in experimental systems (3,4). It was also reasoned that because of the absence of mucositis and marrow suppression with cisplatinum that it could be included to increase intensity of therapy without superimposed extramedullary toxicity. Thus, adding platinum to the above two drugs complimented one of our long-term goals: high-dose intensity allowing myeloid toxicity but not severe overlapping extramedullary toxicity.

Table 1: High-Dose Tandem Combination Chemotherapy

Dose Level		Total Dose After 1 Course	After 2 Courses
1	Cytoxan	4.5g/m²	9 g/m²
	Etoposide	750 mg/m²	1500 mg/m²
	Cisplatinum	120 mg/m²	240 mg/m²
2	Cytoxan	4.5 g/m²	9 g/m²
	Etoposide	900 mg/m²	1800 mg/m²
	Cisplatinum	150 mg/m²	300 mg/m²
3	Cytoxan	5.25 g/m²	10.5 g/m²
	Etoposide	1200 mg/m²	2400 mg/m²
	Cisplatinum	180 mg/m²	360 mg/m²

STUDIES IN BREAST CARCINOMA

From 1985 the emphasis has been on the subgroup of stage IV breast carcinoma with projected short survivals and short disease-free survival (DFS). Patient accrual to this program is still ongoing, we have cautiously escalated this three-drug combination according to the design shown in Table 1 with the intent of determining the maximum tolerated dose (MTD) associated with no life-threatening extramedullary toxicity and no persisting toxicity that would exclude the ability to administer a second HDT. At the same time by randomizing half our patients to "no" marrow infusion we are studying the contribution of ABMT to marrow recovery and disease relapse patterns. The study design is schematically represented in Figure 1. To summarize, patients with stage IV breast cancer Estrogen Receptor Negative (ER-) or Estrogen Receptor Positive (ER+) refractory to hormone therapy were eligible providing the patients had uncontaminated bone marrow by routine histopathologic examination of bone marrow biopsy and adequate vital organ function. Hormone refractory was defined as ER+ with progression on primary hormone therapy (most often Tamoxifen). Patients usually received "induction phase" therapy with Adriamycin and Cyclophosphamide doses of 60 mg/m^2 and 600 mg/m^2 respectively, every 21 days for a median of four cycles. Those patients

DIAGNOSIS: Stage IV Breast Cancer

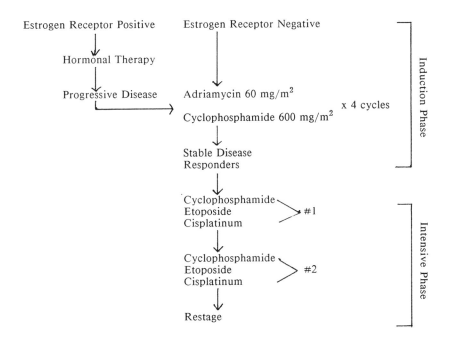

Fig. 1

with stable or responsive disease to induction then enter the "high-dose phase" with Cyclophosphamide, VP-16, and Cisplatinum (CVP), in doses as illustrated in Table 1. Upon completion of one HDT and hematopoietic recovery to greater than 1500 neutrophils/mm^3 and 100,000 platelets/mm^3, patients received a second HDT after approximately a 4-5 week interval. Upon completion of the second HDT patients are clinically restaged. At present we have reached level three of the dose escalation design (see Table 1).

We have treated a total of 63 stage IV breast cancer patients with this therapy. There are 55 patients "first relapse" ER- or ER+ hormonal refractory, 5 patients who were multiple relapse refractory to standard chemotherapy; an additional 2 patients who were first relapse ER+ but not adequately challenged with hormonal therapy to meet criteria of "Tamoxifex failure", and one additional patient who was stage III at diagnosis with ten positive axillary lymph nodes who was rendered no evidence of disease after mastectomy. Patient characteristics are illustrated in Table 2. Sites and number of metastatic sites are illustrated in Table 2. Response will be reported in the homogeneous group of 55 first relapse ER- or ER+ hormonal refractory patients. Toxicity will be reported for all 63 patients.

Induction therapy response was evaluable in only 52 of the 55 ER- or ER+ hormonal refractory patients because 3 were rendered "no evidence of disease" (NED) at the time

Table 2. Patient Characteristics

	ER- or HR* 55 Pts.	Mult.Relapse 5 Pts.	ER+ 2 Pts.	Stage III 1 Pt.
Median Age	43	41	35,45	47
(Range)	(28-62)	(32-54)		
ER Status (%)				
ER-	35 (64)	2 (40)		
ER+	15 (27)	3 (60)	2 (100)	1 (100)
ER?	5 (9)			
Menopausal Status				
Pre	35 (64)	4 (80)	1 (50)	1 (100)
Peri	6 (11)		1 (50)	
Post	14 (25)	1 (20)		
Median Disease-Free				
Interval in Weeks	65	85	56,352	NED**
(Range)	(0-548)	(30-261)		
Sites of Disease (%)				
1 site	18 (33)		2 (100)	NED**
2 sites	16 (29)	2 (40)		
3 sites	12 (22)	3 (60)		
4 sites	7 (13)			
5 sites	2 (3)			

* Hormone Refractory
** No Evidence of Disease, and no recurrent disease at time of high-dose therapy.

they entered induction phase(two with prior local surgical resection and one with prior local radiotherapy). The complete remission rate was 14/52 (27%), and the partial remission was 24/52 (46%). There was an overall response rate (partial and complete) of 38/52 (73%).

The response to the high-dose intensification phase was only evaluable in 35 patients excluding (the 3 NED patients prior to induction, 3 patients who suffered early-death during HDT before response could be evaluated, and 14 additional patients in complete remission after induction phase who were inevaluable for response to the intensive phase). Included in the 14 complete responders to induction is one additional early-death patient who was obviously not evaluable for response to intensive phase, our last early-death patient was a partial responder to induction phase and was included evaluable as a complete responder to intensive phase prior to her death. Our results to intensive phase reveal there was complete remission in 16/35 (46%), and partial remission in 16/35 (46%), for an overall response rate of 32/35 (92%).

Response after completing both phases of induction and intensification in 47 evaluable patients (excluding 5 early deaths and 3 NED patients) was complete remission in 28/47 (60%) and partial remission rate in 16/47 (34%). The overall response rate in patients completing both induction and intensive phases was seen in 44/47 (94%) (Table 3).

Table 3. Response

Responses:	Induction Phase*	Intensive Phase**	After Completing Both Phases***
Complete	14/52 (27%)	16/35 (46%)	28/47 (60%)
Partial	24/52 (46%)	16/35 (46%)	16/47 (34%)
Overall	38/52 (73%)	32/35 (92%)	44/47 (94%)

  * 52 patients evaluable for response at time of induction phase.
 ** 35 patients evaluable for response at time of intensive phase.
*** 47 patients evaluable for response after completing both phases.

The median progression-free survival from induction phase is 58 weeks (53-103) 95% confidence level. The median survival from induction phase is 95 weeks (66-not reached) 95% confidence level. The progression-free survivals and survival compare favorably to ER- cohorts of patients treated with conventional therapy and raises our enthusiasm to continue these studies to generate a sufficient number of patients to more accurately assess if a proportion of patients can be cured from this approach (5,6). Not unexpectedly, patients with less tumor burden (two or fewer sites of metastatic disease) and a longer disease-free interval (DFI greater than 72 weeks) had a longer progression-free survival than other patients in the cohort; these two factors were found to be independent variables.

The major toxicities as expected were infectious; 38% sepsis during cycle one and 46% during cycle 2. There is an 11% incidence of pneumonia during cycle one and 7% incidence during cycle 2. Ninety per cent of our patients experienced a fever greater than 100.4° F. during each cycle with a median duration of 5 and 8 days respectively. Among the total of 63 patients treated there were five deaths 5/63 (8%). Four of these deaths are due to infection (three bacterial sepsis , one fungal sepsis) and one secondary to myocardial infarction.

Marrow infusion did significantly enhance platelet recovery, but only helped neutrophil recovery marginally. During the second cycle we observed late recovery of hematopoietic elements in 25% of cases randomized to the no marrow infusion arm, but differences were not of sufficient clinical difference to terminate the randomization.

PRESENT PERSPECTIVE

Our impressive complete remission rates are equivalent to most other reported studies using HDT with ABMT (7). To evaluate the full potential of this program, we have to determine if a plateau exists in the progression-free survival curve. If we can detect a definite small plateau, this would support the concept of potential cure using this approach in the treatment of metastatic breast cancer. The double HDT approach allows some flexibility such as the introduction of an alternative non-cross-resistant combination in the second high-dose treatment position. Further modifications could include more selective eligibility administering this double therapy to only the prognostic-favorable subgroup who are responsive to induction, while developing alternate more aggressive approaches to the prognostic-unfavorable subgroup of patients not achieving response to induction therapy. Innovative use of growth factors and other maneuvers to attempt to ameliorate duration of neutropenia will aid in removing our major toxicity (infection). Since we have not reached the maximum tolerated dose, careful dose escalation is warranted in an attempt to exploit the dose intensity curve achieving maximal tumor kill while remaining below the critical threshold at which prohibitive extramedullary toxicity is encountered (8).

This approach has promise for use in the group of high-risk stage III breast cancer patients. Patients with inflammatory breast cancer and locally advanced breast cancer have a poor prognoses when treated with local regional therapy alone. It is this group of patients with minimal microscopic residual disease which may benefit most from high-dose consolidation therapy after completion of their neo-adjuvant and local/regional therapy.

The question of marrow contamination is still not resolved. It is conceivable that in the arm randomized to marrow infusion some patients may be given occult tumor cells at the time of marrow reinfusion. Whether or not these tumor cells will be able to establish recurrent metastatic disease, or influence marrow recovery patterns, is still undetermined. It is conceivable that differences in relapse patterns could only be critically compared in those patients achieving complete remission and maintaining prolonged disease-free survival before they develop clinically detectable new tumor masses. New, more sensitive detection methods for occult marrow or circulating peripheral tumor cells are on the horizon to study this phenomenon (9).

IMMEDIATE FUTURE DIRECTIONS

Future directions include the development of an alternate combination of drugs which is non-cross resistant with the cyclophosphamide, etoposide, cisplatinum (CVP) combination, this may be useful especially if after achieving maximum tolerated dose of our CVP program we do not achieve a gratifying enough number of long-term disease-free survivors statistically superior to conventional chemotherapy. An alternate combination may also be useful in those prognostically unfavorable patients which are progressing after induction therapy (a group for which our double cisplatinum approach seems to have only transient effect at the present doses). In an attempt to reduce our major toxicity (infection) which is secondary to duration of neutropenia we are actively investigating peripheral blood stem cell collection, autologous bone marrow collection, and reinfusion of both products in combination with recombinate growth factors. If we can reduce the duration of neutropenia by these maneuvers we anticipate our major toxicity (infection) would be eliminated.

REFERENCES

1. Farha P, Spitzer G, Valdivieso M., Dicke KA, Zander AR, Dhingra HM, Minnhaar G, Vellekoop L, Verma DS, Umsawasadi T: High-dose chemotherapy and autologous bone marrow transplantation for the treatment of small cell lung carcinoma. Cancer 52:1351-1355, 1983.
2. Spitzer G, Farha P, Valdivieso M, Dicke K, Zander A, Vellekoop L, Murphy WK, Dhingra HM, Umsawsadi T, Chiuten D, Carr DT: High-dose intensification therapy with autologous bone marrow support for limited small-cell bronchogenic carcinoma. J Clin Oncol 1986;4:4-13.
3. Forastiere A, Hakes T: Cisplatinum in the treatment of metastatic breast carcinoma. Am J Clin Oncol 1982; 5:243
4. Kolaric K, Roth A: Phase II clinical trial of cis-dichlorodiamine platinum (cis-DDP) for antitumorigenic activity in previously untreated patients with metastatic breast cancer. Cancer Chemother Pharmacol II:108-112,1983.
5. Kiang D, Gay J: A randomized trial of chemotherapy and hormonal therapy in advanced breast cancer. New Engl J Med 1985; 313:1241-46.
6. Mortimer J, Livingston R: Aggressive Doxorubicin-Containing Regimen (Prednisone, Methotrexate, 5-FU, Doxorubricin, and Cyclophosphamide; PM-FAC) in Disseminated Estrogen Receptor-Negative Breast Cancer. Cancer Treatment Reports Vol 68, No 7-8. July/Aug. 1984.
7. Peters W, Shpall E: High-dose combination alkylating agents with bone marrow support as initial treatment for metastatic breast cancer. J Clin Oncol 1988; 6:1368-76.
8. Henderson I, Hayes F: Dose-response in the treatment of breast cancer: A critical review. J Clin Oncol 1988; 6:1501-15.
9. Taha M, Ordoñez NG, Kulkarni S, Owen M, Hortobagyi G, Reading CL, Dicke KA, Spitzer G: A monoclonal antibody cocktail for detection of micrometastatic tumor cells in the bone marrow of breast cancer patients. Bone Marrow Transplantation 1989 (in press).

12

MAMMARY CARCINOGENESIS

J. RUSSO AND I.H. RUSSO

Department of Pathology, Michigan Cancer Foundation, 110 East
Warren Avenue, Detroit, MI 48201

INTRODUCTION

Breast cancer incidence is increasing in tne western world.
Despite of considerable advances in detection and treatment, we
seem to be unable to stop the hundred of thousands of new cases
diagnosed every passing year. Our failure to control this disease
is basically rooted in our lack of knowledge of the biology of
breast cancer.

There are many questions that need to be answered in order to
understand the biology of breast cancer (1), however there are
four basic ones that will be the subject of this work. They are:
what causes breast cancer?; how does breast cancer start?; what
are the determinants of the susceptibility of the gland to
carcinogenesis?, what determines that an initiated cell progresses
to a fully malignant one, and lastly, can breast cancer be
prevented?

We do not know what the etiological factors are, the only
tning that we know is that several risk factors are related to
breast cancer (1-4). Among them we know that women are more prone
to develop breast cancer than men (1,4). Breast cancer is
diagnosed more frequently in women over 40 years of age, even
though a trend to increased incidence in younger patients has been
observed (1,4,5). Women witn family history of breast cancer have
a 9:1 greater chance to develop the disease (4,6). The presence
of premalignant lesions is also associated with higher risk (1-4)
and lastly, it nas been shown that reproductive history has a
significant weight in the risk to develop breast cancer (1,3,6-8).

134

EXPERIMENTAL SYSTEMS

These observations suggest that in order to understand how
these factors affect the biology of the disease and how they can
be manipulated, an adequate experimental system is needed (1).
The experimental system that we have used in our study is that
developed by Huggins (9), and consists in the inoculation of the
polycyclic hydrocarbon 7,12-dimethylbenz(a)anthracene (DMBA) to
virgin Sprague Dawley rats, which is a strain of animals highly
susceptible to develop chemically-induced carcinomas.

In this model, the intragastric administration of carcinogen
to young but sexually mature virgin animals of approximately 55
days-of-age induces up to 100% tumor incidence. Endocrine
manipulation and diet are important factors in the overall tumor
incidence. Studies utilizing the direct acting carcinogen
N-methyl-N-nitrosourea (NMU) have shown similar characteristics in
tumor development (9-12).

PATHOGENESIS OF MAMMARY CARCINOMA

Mammary cancer results from the interaction of two basic
components, the carcinogen and the target organ (1). The
carcinogen in our experimental system is known, and the target
organ is obviously the mammary gland. The mammary gland, however,
does not respond as a unit to the carcinogenic insult. The fact
that it is composed of a complex branching system requires to
identify within this complexity the target site for carcinogenic
initiation. We have been able to identify the terminal end bud
(TEB) as the site of origin of mammary carcinomas (13-15). The
TEB is the primitive element of the gland that at the time of
puberal growth in the rat (at about 25-35 days of age) they start
to bifurcate into alveolar buds (ABs); these, with successive
estrous cycles progress to virginal lobules (14-17). If the
carcinogen is given at this time of active differentiation of TEBs
to ABs, within 14 days of carcinogen administration the first
lesions are observed at the level of one or various adjacent TEBs,
which show enlargement and a more dark appearance in the whole
mount preparation (14,16). These lesions are called intraductal

proliferations or IDPs (14,16). IDPs are easily distinguished from the gland's normal ductal structures by the presence of a multilayered epithelium (14,16,18). Lesions arising in adjacent TEBs tend to coalesce forming microtumors, which become evident after 20 days of DMBA administration (16). Both microtumors and palpable tumors are in general adenocarcinomas with solid, cribriform or papillary patterns. They are composed of epithelial cells characterized by nuclear pleomorphism, increased nuclear size and moderate mitotic activity (16). When the tumors progress, they invade the stroma forming the typical infiltrating ductal carcinoma (19). If the animal is allowed to live long enough, metastases occur, mainly to the lungs (19).

The mammary gland affected by the carcinogen develops benign lesions as well. Hyperplastic lobules, showing secretory activity appear in moderate numbers, and later than IDPs. Adenomas, fibroadenomas and cysts are seen scattered throughout the glands.

The transformation of terminal end buds to intraductal proliferations is the first event in carcinogenesis, being observed as early as 14 day post-carcinogen administration, whereas benign lesions such as fibroadenomas, cysts and hyperplastic lobules appear later. We postulate that there is a different pathogenetic pathway for benign and malignant rat mammary tumors. The TEB is the site of origin of carcinomas, whereas benign lesions such as alveolar hyperplasias, cysts, adenomas, and fibroadenomas are originated from more differentiated structures such as ABs and primitive lobules (Fig. 1). The fact that benign lesions tend to appear later than the malignant ones indicates that the former are not precursors of the latter (1,11,12).

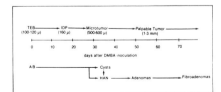

Figure 1: Chart representing the pathogenetic pathway of malignant lesions. The affected terminal end bud (TEB) originates an intraductal proliferation (I.D.P.) and this progresses to carcinoma in situ, developing in time various patterns. (Reprinted with permission from ref 1).

PROGRESSION OF INITIATED CELLS TO CARCINOMA

We have observed that the earliest event in mammary carcinogenesis is the transformation of TEBs into IDPs, which progressively evolve to carcinomas (Fig 1).

IDPs are morphologically distinguishable from TEBs by their size, that is more then twice that of the TEB and by the homogenous cell composition, which consists preponderantly of intermediate cells (1,11,20). As it is depicted in Figure 2 the induction of IDPs is by no means a rare event. Within three weeks of DMBA administration there are around 20 IDPs per gland, and this number increases with time, such that by 6 to 10 weeks after treatment there are approximately 30 lesions per gland, and around 200 per animal. Although IDPs occur in large numbers following DMBA administration, the likelihood of any one IDP of progressing to carcinoma in the intact mammary gland is lower than that, since the maximal tumorigenic response rarely goes beyond 5 to 6

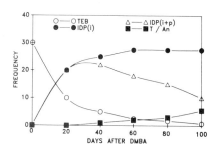

Figure 2: Emergence of preneoplastic lesions. Intraductal proliferation (IDP)-initiated IDP (i), initiated and promoted-IDP (i+p), increase by 20 days post-DMBA. IDPs (i+p) decrease as they progress to carcinomas, expressed as number of tumors per animal (T/An) (From: Russo, J., Russo, I.H., In: Boundaries in mammary Carcinogenesis. O. Sudilovsky (ed.) Plenum Publishing Corp. (1989) (with permission).

adenocarcinomas per animal (Fig. 2). This is attributed to the fact that there are two different types of IDP, one that we call "initiated" IDP, "IDP (i)", whose number increases steadily, with a concomitant decrease in the number of TEBs, but they reach a plateau by 60 days post-DMBA (Fig. 2). The IDP (i) is characterized by having a diameter larger than that of the TEB, and being composed of a greater number of epithelial cells. They do not elicit a response in the surrounding stroma, and remain unchanged during the whole post carcinogen observation period. A second type of IDP, that we call "initiated and promoted" "IDP (i+p)" arises at the same time and reaches the same level than IDPs (i); by 20 to 30 days post-DMBA they are also characterized by having a larger diameter and a greater cell number than TEBs as well, but they elicit a marked stromal reaction, consisting in collagen deposition and infiltration by mast cells and lymphocytes. IDPs (i+p) progress to carcinoma in situ and to invasive carcinoma (Fig. 2). The fact that not all the IDPs progress to carcinoma indicates that although both IDPs (i) and (i+p) are preneoplastic lesions, there are factors that regulate the progression of initiated cells, which affect differently IDPs (i) and IDPs (i+p).

The factors that regulate the progression of an initiated cell to preneoplasia and to neoplasia are unknown, however, we have been able to identify a host response elicited by the initiated cells that might play a role in this mechanism. This host response consists in infiltration of the stroma surrounding the IDP by mast cells. The number of mast cells around the IDP (i+p) is three times higher than in TEBs and IDP (i). This increase in mast cells is accompanied by an increase in lymphocytes, fibroblasts, collagen fibers and proteoglycans.

Mast cells are found in different parts of the body, and the mammary gland is not an exception. They contain in their cytoplasm numerous granules, that stain metachromatically with toluidine blue or alcian blue (21). These granules measure up to 0.8 um in diameter (21). Mast cells have membrane receptors to IgE that participate in the immediate and delayed type of hypersensitivity (22). When an antigen combines with IgE and binds the cell receptor, the cell degranulates releasing histamine and heparin. Heparin is a heparan sulfate that has shown to stimulate cell proliferation (23). It has been shown that transplanted tumors in the chick embryo may increase by 40 fold the number of mast cells around the tumor implant before new capillaries arise (24). Mast cell lysates or mast cell-conditioned medium stimulate locomotion of capillary endothelial cells in vitro (25,26), an effect that is attributed to heparin. It has been postulated that heparin or fragments of heparin on the surface of endothelial cells may selectively bind endothelial cell mitogens that are also angiogenic

138

(23). Interestingly enough there are several growth factors that
have great affinity for heparin (27,28). It has also been shown
that heparin-coated tumor cells exhibit altered transplantation and
cytotoxicity reaction (29,30), presumably due to blockage of cell
surface antigens by heparin. Thus, heparan sulfate proteoglycans
also may be deposited in an annulus around the tumor and may
modulate the immunoreactivity or accessibility of the enclosed
cells.

An early change observed during the process of transformation
is the synthesis of a large amount of proteoglycans by IDP (i+p)
which is evidenced by the deposition of an electron dense material
on the cell surface of the epithelial cells, and by increased
reactivity with alcian blue pH 2.7 and PAS. This is accompanied by
an increase in uptake of 3H-fucose and 3H-glucosamine (Fig. 3).
The number of cells uptaking these precursors is almost three times
the number found in TEBs and IDPs (i) (Fig. 3). These data clearly
indicate that the initiated cells that are progressing to
malignancy are secreting proteoglycans that start to accumulate in
the stroma. We do not know if these proteoglycans secreted by the
epithelial cells are influencing the response of the host by
eliciting a higher mobilization of mast cells inhibiting the
cytotoxic effect of lymphocytes, or inducing angiogenesis,
desmoplasia or cell proliferation. Some of these proteoglycans,
such as heparan sulfate, act as receptors for growth factors, which
in turn initiate an autocrine response.

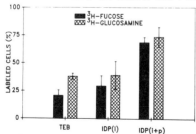

Figure 3: Histogram showing the
percentage of cells labeled with
3H-fucose and 3H-glucosamine in
TEB, IDP(i) and IDP(i+p). From:
Russo, J, Russo, I.H., In:
Boundaries in Mammary
Carcinogenesis. O. Sudilovsky (ed.)
Plenum Publishing Corp. (1989) (with
permission).

Proteoglycans occur on the plasma membranes of mammalian cells
and in the extracellular matrix (31-33). They are of two types: i)
neutral glycoproteins that are stained by PAS, are negative with
alcian blue pH 2.7 and contain fucose residues; ii) acid

mucopolysaccharides, which react with alcian blue pH 2.7 and react
negatively with PAS; these in turn, are of two types:
glycosaminoglycans of chondroitin sulfate, containing residues of
D-glucuronic acid and N-acetyl-D- galactosamine and
glycosaminoglycans of heparan sulfate, which contain alternating
residues of D-glucuronic acid or L-iduronic acid and N-acetyl-D-
glucosamine.

Neoplastic transformation of cells dramatically alters
proteoglycan synthesis both in the tumor and in the surrounding
tissue (34). This alteration in proteoglycan synthesis is thought
to stimulate tumorigenic growth by decreasing the adhesion of
transformed cells to the extracellular matrix (35).

Based upon our own data and in those reported in the
literature, it is possible to speculate that the production of
proteoglycans allows the IDP to progress to carcinoma in situ by
stimulation of cell proliferation and by interference with an
immune reaction toward the cells. Of these newly synthesized
proteoglycans both, those that incorporate 3H-D-glucosamine and
stain with alcian blue pH 2.7 and those that uptake 3H-fucose and
stain with PAS may act like epiglycanin, a high molecular weight
sialoglycoprotein present in mouse mammary carcinoma (Ta3) cells,
which is thought to mask histocompatibility antigens (36). These
in turn, can prevent the generation and penetration of cytolytic
lymphocytes (29).

MODULATION OF MAMMARY GLAND SUSCEPTIBILITY TO CARCINOGENESIS.

During the postnatal development of the mammary gland, the
number of TEBs reaches a peak in the 21 day-old female and then
they start to reduce both in size and number due to their
differentiation into ABs and lobules (14,15). Being the TEB the
site of origin of mammary carcinomas, it is possible to predict
that carcinogen inoculation at various times during the lifespan of
a virgin animal will result in an incidence of carcinomas
proportional to the number of TEBs. This was observed to be true.
The older the animal at the time of carcinogen administration, the
fewer the number of tumors developed (1,13). It was also

observed that not all the mammary glands responded to the administration of the carcinogen in the same fashion; tumor incidence in
thoracic mammary glands was higher than in the abdominal mammary
glands (1,17,20). This different carcinogenic response is due to the
asynchronous development of glands located in different topographic
areas; thoracic glands lag behind in development and retain a higher
concentration of TEBs (1,20). This asynchrony reduces with aging, and
the thoracic glands approach the degree of development of glands seen
in other locations; by the age of 330 days tumor incidence is similar
in both glands located in either a thoracic or abdominal region (20).

A further evidence in support of the TEB as the site of origin of
mammary carcinomas has been obtained by plotting the incidence of
adenocarcinomas, or percentage of animals bearing this tumor type
against the percentage of TEBs present in the mammary gland at the
time of carcinogen administration. A high correlation coefficient (CR
= 0.83, p   0.001) between these two parameters has been observed.
However, there is no correlation between tumor incidence and the
number of other terminal structures such as ABs or lobules (20).

Further evidence that it is the number of TEBs which affects the
susceptibility of the mammary gland to carcinogenesis is obtained
through the study of pregnancy. Full term pregnancy, that completely
eliminates TEBs also results in inhibition of tumor development in
parous animals (Fig. 4) (1,11,37-39). If pregnancy is interrupted,
however, this protection is minimized or nullified (Fig. 4) (40).
Hormonal manipulation with estrogenic compounds (20,41-44) or with
chorionic gonadotropin (1,20,45) demonstrates that reductions in
number of TEBs similar to those occurring after pregnancy can be
induced by these treatments, thus resulting in different degrees of
refractoriness (1).

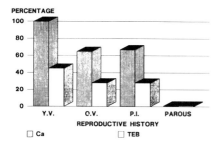

Figure 4: Correlation between
incidence of DMBA-induced
adenocarcinomas (Ca) and percentage
of TEBs (ordinate) in young virgin
(Y.V.), old (O.V.), pregnancy
interruption (P.I.) and parous rats
(abscissa). (Reprinted with
permission from ref. 20)

One of the elements that influence the susceptibility of the TEB to carcinogenesis is the high proliferative activity of its epithelium (1,46,47). We have measured the growth fraction of TEBs; we found that their proliferative compartment is the highest among all structures of the mammary gland. Fifty five percent of the cells are proliferating in the TEB of virgin rats, whereas only 23% are in the proliferative pool in ABs and lobules (47). The growth fraction decreases with both aging and differentiation (47). In the gland of parous animals, which is refractory to carcinogenesis, the growth fraction is only 1% (47).

Cells of the TEBs cycle approximately every 10 hours, with an S phase of about 7 hours and a G1 or resting phase of one hour (47). When the mammary gland is differentiated by pregnancy, the growth fraction is reduced about 60 times and the cells that are proliferating have a cell cycle lengthened to about 35 hours. This lengthening occurs at the expense of the G1 phase of the cell cycle (1,47). Therefore, pregnancy shifts the cells to a resting compartment.

Carcinogenic initiation requires the stable alteration of DNA molecules (1,11). For this the carcinogen has to bind to the DNA, and maximal DNA binding occurs when a peak of maximal DNA synthesis is taking place in the organ. Carcinogens damage DNA mostly during the S-phase (48-51). If the damage is not repaired during the G1 phase, the damaged DNA is transmitted to the daughter cells and it becomes fixed during successive S-phases of the cycle (48-51). We have demonstrated that the uptake of tritiated DMBA is selectively higher in TEBs than in other structures of the mammary gland; this uptake, expressed as the number of grains per nucleus, highly correlates with the DNA synthetic activity of the cells or DNA-LI (11).

DMBA is metabolized by the mammary epithelium to both polar and phenolic metabolites. The metabolic pathway is similar in both the TEBs of virgin rats and the lobules of parous animals, however, the formation of polar metabolites is higher in the TEB epithelial cells, and the binding of the carcinogen to DNA is also higher in these cells than in lobular cells (1,52,53). Adduct removal from the DNA has also a different pattern. TEBs have a very low rate of adduct removal, whereas lobules are more efficient, indicating that these latter structures repair the damage induced by the carcinogen more efficiently (45,53).

HORMONE PREVENTION OF MAMMARY CARCINOGENESIS

Experimentally induced breast cancer (9-11) is prevented if the animal undergoes a full-term pregnancy prior to exposure to a given carcinogen (10-12,54-56), or by administration of exogenous hormones such as chorionic gonadotropin (38,57), estrogens and progesterone, either alone or in combination (58,59), pituitary homografts (58), or contraceptive agents (41-43,60,61). An understanding of how hormones modulate the susceptibility of this organ to carcinogenesis has been achieved through the knowledge of the pathogenesis of chemically induced mammary carcinomas (13-15). The demonstration in the 7,12-dimethylbenz(a)anthracene (DMBA) induced-rat mammary carcinoma model that the presence of undifferentiated structures or TEBs determines mammary cancer incidence (11,12,14,15,62), and that full differentiation of the gland induced by pregnancy eliminates the targets of the carcinogen, clearly indicate that differentiation plays a key role in carcinogenesis, mainly because it reduces the high cell proliferative activity observed in the TEB (11,12). Differentiation also shifts the cells from the proliferating to the resting compartment, the DMBA-DNA binding is significantly reduced, the DNA repair is more efficient and the cells produce less polar metabolites (11), all biological parameters that determine the susceptibility of the mammary gland to carcinogenesis. Cell proliferation is of importance because carcinogens induce a greater oncogenic response in dividing than in non dividing cells (48,49) and maximal sensitivity to transformation occurs in the late G_1 or S phases of the cell cycle (50,51). It is therefore reasonable to assume that hormonally induced changes in the architecture of the gland and in the cell kinetic properties of the epithelium modulate its susceptibility to carcinogenesis. This concept suggests that induction of gland differentiation early enough in

life, before the mammary epithelium is altered in its ability to
undergo normal development or is exposed to a carcinogenic stimulus
is probably the most physiological approach to breast cancer
prevention (13,41-44,56), since this mechanism inhibits initiation
of the process by eliminating the undifferentiated terminal ductal
structures that are the target of the carcinogen (14,15,39,44).
Protection of the mammary gland by modifying its structure under
controlled circumstances is a pressing issue, especially in the
western world, where women are increasingly entering the high risk
pool, which can be defined as: early menarche (63,64), late parity
or nulliparity (4,6), and exogenous hormone usage (64) among other
factors (3,7,8,65).

Use of Estrogenic and Progestagenic Agents in Breast Cancer
Prevention

Since mammary gland development and differentiation are under
the control of ovarian hormones, with oestrogens stimulating growth
of the mammary epithelium (66) and progesterone determining the
formation of alveoli (67), we tested the ability of the most
commonly utilized combination of oestrogens and progestagens,
contraceptive agents, in inducing mammary gland differentiation
(2,60,68,69).

Although oral contraceptives have been widely studied, their
effect on mammary gland development and cancer remains
controversial, and their mechanism of action is not completely
understood. Our results show that there are numerous variables that
have to be carefully balanced to achieve the desired effects, and
that contraceptive use in nulliparous females can become a
two-edged sword, depending upon the type of hormone and dose used.
We utilized the following experimental protocol: four groups of 75
virgin female Sprague-Dawley rats, were treated when they reached
the ages of 45, 55, 65 or 75 days with a pellet implanted
subcutaneously. The pellets contained: a) Norethynodrel (98.5%)
-mestranol (1.5%) (NM), or b) medroxyprogesterone acetate (MPA)
(Innovative Research of America, Rockville, MD), both at two doses:
a physiological dose, (low dose-LD) (NM.LD) or (MPA.LD),
administered in 0.5 mg pellets, a dose that was estimated to be

equivalent to the that used by women with the purpose of
contraception (70), and 5.0 mg pellets or high dose (NM.HD or
MPA.HD), which was a ten fold increase above the physiological
dose.

Norethynodrel-Mestranol as a Hormone-Preventive Agent

Our results demonstrated that a 21-day treatment of virgin rats
with the combined estrogenic-progestagenic agent
norethynodrel-mestranol terminated 21 days prior to exposure to
DMBA, had a protective effect against the subsequent development of
tumors in general and against adenocarcinomas in particular. This
protective effect was attributed to the influence of the hormones
on mammary gland structure, since a significant correlation between
reduction in the percentage of TEBs in the mammary gland and
incidence of adenocarcinomas was found. A similar protective
effect from chemical carcinogenesis has been reported in rats
treated with estrogenic hormones and progesterone prior to DMBA or
NMU administration (59,71). Although a protective effect of Enovid
has been reported (2,41,42,60), Welsch and Meites (60) found that
its administration to rats starting 25 days before and continuing
for 15 days after DMBA inoculation reduced the number of tumors per
animal and lengthened the latency period, But without affecting
overall tumor incidence.

The precise mechanisms by which norethynodrel-mestranol exerts
a protective effect remain to be elucidated, but it is logical to
assume that the observed morphological and cell kinetic changes
induced by this hormone combination treatment in the mammary gland
modify the cell's ability to metabolize, bind and/or remove adducts
or repair damage induced by carcinogen treatment, factors that have
been shown to play a role in the protection mediated by pregnancy
(1,12,53).

In our experiments, we challenged with a carcinogen a mammary
epithelium that had returned to a quiescent condition after
hormonal stimulation. This indicates that treatment resulted in
permanent changes which affected tumor initiation by decreasing the
number of target structures (1,9,11-16,45,56,72).

Although norethynodrel is related to 19-nortestosterone, it is

a weak progestagen and induces a low maximal McPnail index,
inducing perinuclear vacuolization in endometrial cells, being in
this respect more similar to estrone than to progesterone (73).
The influence of this hormone combined with mestranol on, body
weight, mammary gland development, and tumor incidence, appears to
be associated witn its predominant estrogenic action. It remains
to be elucidated whether estrogenic contraceptives have some direct
effect on the mammary epithelium, as has been demonstrated for
17-B-estradiol in the mouse (66), and human (74,75), or whether
they act indirectly decreasing the hypothalamic content of
prolactin inhibiting factor and increasing pituitary prolactin
concentration (60,73) or through other endocrine regulatory
mechanisms. This hormone combination diminishes significantly the
number of TEBs, furthering their development to TDs and/or ABs,
depending upon the age at which they are administered. The
diminution in the number of TEBs that are the targets of the
carcinogen correlates with tne decreased number of adenocarcinomas
developed, however, at difference of full-term pregnancy (76), the
protection induced by NM is less efficient, what could be explained
by its inability to completely differentiate the mammary gland.
This indicates that otner hormones, in addition of estrogen and
progesterone, are important in inducing full differentiation of
this organ (1,2,11,38,76-78).

Oral contraceptive use by women is generally accepted to reduce
the risk of both fibroadenoma and benign breast disease
development, but only if in tne latter epithelial atypia is minimal
or absent (79-82), the degree of protection increasing with time of
usage (82-85). These epidemiologic observations are confirmed in
our experimental model, in which treated animals developed fewer
benign lesions, namely fibroadenomas and lactating adenomas, in
addition to the reduction in adenocarcinomas. Although in humans
the role of oral contraceptives on the risk of developing breast
cancer is still controversial, most authors consider that they have
no influence on breast cancer risk (83,85-88) and have no adverse
effect on breast cancer prognosis (84-88).

Our studies allowed us to conclude that treatment with the

combination contraceptive norethynodrel-mestranol prior to administration of the chemical carcinogen DMBA exerts a protective influence from neoplastic transformation, which is measurable as permanent changes in mammary gland structure. The degree of protection is related to dose, and there exists a trend, though not significant, to produce less effect when treatment is initiated at a later age.

Influence of Medroxyprogesterone Acetate on Mammary Carcinogenesis

We observed that treatment with medroxyprogesterone acetate (MPA) at the dose clinically used for contraception in Depo-Provera (70) affected the mammary gland structure and its tumorigenic response differently than treatment with a 10 fold higher or pharmacologic dose. MPA.LD resulted in statistically significant reduction in percentage of TEBs only in animals whose treatment started at age 55, which correlated with the observed lower tumor and adenocarcinoma incidence. However, low dose treatment initiated at all the other ages did not modify the probability of a rat developing a tumor. Rats treated with the high dose on the other hand, were 2.45 times more likely to develop a tumor than controls. Both doses resulted in a higher percentage of TEBs in animals treated at ages older tnan 65. These results contrasted markedly with those observed in rats treated with both low and high dose norethynodrel-mestranol (2,43) in which the hormonal treatment resulted in a dose dependent significant reduction in percentage of TEBs and reduction in the incidence of DMBA-induced both tumors and adenocarcinomas. A protective effect of ovarian hormones has been reported by various authors (60,69,71). Huggins et al., (9) observed that 17B-estradiol had a protective effect when given in combination with progesterone, decreasing cancer incidence when the hormones were administered 15 days post-DMBA instillation, whereas pregnancy and progesterone alone accelerated tumor growth. Increased tumor incidence as a consequence of progestagenic hormonal treatment has been reported in other species such as beagle dogs, which develop malignant and metastatic mammary tumors after treatment with low and high doses of depot MPA (89-91). In Balb/c mice, depot MPA treatment induces a high incidence of invasive mammary adenocarcinomas (92,93).

These studies, however, attest of the carcinogenic effect of the hormone per se; ours is the first study that reports the influence of MPA on mammary gland structure prior to exposure to DMBA, thus acting as a modifier of the response of this organ to a chemical carcinogen. The effect of both MPA.LD and HD on mammary gland structure was manifested in the 75 day-old animals as an inhibition of mammary gland differentiation, namely inhibition of the progression of TEBs to ABs, and of these to lobules, which resulted in a relative increase in the number of TEBs over the number normally found in age-matched animals. These structural changes had a statistically significant correlation with the incidence of adenocarcinomas developed after exposure to carcinogen. In those groups in which a significant increment in number of TEBs was observed there was an inverse correlation with number of TDs and of ABs. It remains to be elucidated whether the effect of this acetoxyprogesterone derivative, which is qualitatively similar, but more potent than progesterone (73) on mammary gland development, is mediated by its progestagenic, androgenic or synandrogenic effects (94).

In the DMBA rat mammary carcinoma model, progesterone, like estradiol, when administered during the latent period following DMBA, reduced the latency period and increased the size and number of tumors developed (95-97), although progesterone does not maintain hormone dependent carcinomas in castrated rats.

In humans, the role of progesterone is elusive. It has been reported that luteal phase plasma progesterone levels are significantly reduced in women with benign breast disease (98), and progesterone deficiency has been considered to be associated with greater breast cancer risk in premenopausal patients (99). England, et al (100), on the other hand, reported that women with cystic disease have elevated luteal progesterone, and elevated levels of progesterone have also been detected in daughters of breast cancer patients (101,102). Progesterone and progestagens are used therapeutically, since, when given in pharmacological amounts, cause regression in hormone-dependent neoplasias of the endometrium (103).

The possible role of progestagenic contraceptives in the etiology of breast cancer is far from being clarified. Nevertheless, epidemiologic studies have linked the use of high progestagen contraceptive agents to a higher risk of developing cervical cancer (85) and when administered before a full term pregnancy, to higher risk of breast cancer (104,105). However, epidemiologic observations in general tend to consider that combination oral contraceptives have no influence on breast cancer risk (98,106-108); these findings are confirmed by our results showing that the combination compound norethyndrel- mestranol, which in the rat is mostly estrogenic, has a protective effect from chemically induced carcinogenesis, whereas the progestagenic compound MPA tends to increase tumor incidence (2,41-44,60,69). Therefore, our studies allowed us to conclude that in the DMBA-rat mammary gland system, MPA treatment at the dose used for contraception did not significantly affect mammary gland development, and therefore did not modify the response of the organ to the administration of a chemical carcinogen, whereas a 10 fold increase in dose resulted in inhibition of gland differentiation in the group treated at 75 days of age, with an increase in number of targets and a consequent increase in tumor incidence.

Influence of Hormonal Treatment on the Risk to Develop Carcinomas

Evaluation of tumor incidence in terms of relative risk (RR), or ratio between incidence of adenocarcinomas observed in experimental and in control animals, in which an incidence of carcinomas equal to the control was 1, it was observed that NM.LD reduced tumor incidence and therefore RR to 0.66, 0.37 and 0.24 in the groups treated at 45, 55 and 65 days of age, respectively, but no protective effect was seen when treatment was initiated at 75 days of age, since in this group RR was 1.0 (Fig. 5). NM.HD showed to be more protective in all ages administered, since animals thus treated had RR of 0.31, 0.13, 0.37 and 0.56 when treatments were initiated at the same ages. MPA, on the other hand, reduced the risk only when administered at either LD or HD to animals aged 55 or 65 days, whereas administration to 45 day-old animals increased the risk to 1.09 and 1.19 for the LD and HD respectively, and to 1.95 when administered at either LD or HD to 75-day-old animals (Fig. 5).

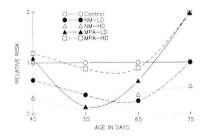

Figure 5: Relative risk (ordinate) or ratio between DMBA-induced mammary adenocarcinomas developed by NM.LD, NM.HD, MPA.LD adn MPA.HD treated rats and controls (RR=1). (Reprinted with permission from ref. 20).

Use of the Placental Hormone Chorionic Gonadotropin in Breast Cancer Prevention.

Since we know that pregnancy protects the mammary gland from DMBA-induced carcinogenesis, and the main placental hormone is chorionic gonadotropin, we felt that the most rational hormone to test in protecting the mammary gland through differentiation will be this placental hormone (1).

Based upon this rationale, we inoculated for 21 days various doses of pure chorionic gonadotropin to virgin females, then the animals were allowed to rest for 21 days and then they received DMBA. We found that treatment with 1-10 IU of chorionic gonadotropin (hCG) produced a significant protection of the mammary gland, but complete protection, meaning no carcinoma development, occurred when 100 IU were given to the animals. This treatment also reduced the number of TEBs and the rate of DNA-synthesis in the mammary gland (1).

In in vitro experiments measuring the rate of DMBA adduct removal by epithelial cells of young virgin, old virgin and parous animals, it was observed that cells treated with chorionic gonadotropin had an enhanced rate of adduct removal to a greater degree than even full-term pregnancy (1).

Chorionic gonadotropin protects the mammary gland through induction of full differentiation, induction of depression of DNA synthesis, inhibition of the binding of the carcinogen to DNA and an increase of the ability of the cells to repair the damaged DNA (1,45). We concluded that chorionic gonadotropin treatment is, with a full-term pregnancy the most physiological means for preventing breast cancer.

SUMMARY AND CONCLUSIONS

Through the study of mammary carcinomas induced by the inoculation of the polycyclic hydrocarbon 7,12-dimethylbenz(a)anthracene (DMBA) to young virgin Sprague-Dawley rats it has been determined that carcinogenic initiation occurs only when undifferentiated terminal ductal structures or terminal end buds (TEBs) are present in the mammary gland. Tumor incidence is modulated by variations in the number of these structures, as their reduction with aging or their total disappearance with full-term pregnancy results in either marked diminution or abolition of neoplastic transformation. The high susceptibility of the TEB to neoplastic transformation is due to its high mitotic activity, short cell cycle, resulting in fixation of transformation, and inefficient DNA repair. Transformed TEBs progress to intraductal proliferations (IDPs) and these to carcinomas which become invasive and eventually metastatic. DMBA also induces benign lesions which result from transformation of more differentiated structures such as alveolar buds (ABs) and lobules. The progression of IDP to carcinoma seems to be mediated by specific host's reactions, namely mast cell and lymphocytic infiltration, as well as by increased synthesis of proteoglycans by transformed cells. The protective effect induced by pregnancy led to test hormonally-induced differentiating prior to carcinogen administration with the purpose of protection. An estrogenic-progestagenic combination and chorionic gonadotropin exert a powerful differentiating and protective effect from neoplastic transformation, whereas the progestagenic agent medroxyprogesterone acetate tends to induce no protection or to increase breast cancer risk.

Finally, regardless of whether these hormones could be used in humans to prevent the initiation of breast cancer, it is important to bear in mind that it is necessary to know what is the sequence in which the hormones reach their target. If the hormonal stimulus reaches a TEB that has been already affected by a carcinogen, these hormones will act on cells initiated in the neoplastic process, and they might act as promotors of tumorigenesis. If the hormones, on

the other hand, reach a normal TEB, they will induce
differentiation, thus eliminating the possible targets of
carcinogens and abolishing the potential of the gland for
neoplastic transformation.

REFERENCES
1. Russo, J. and Russo, I.H. Lab. Invest. 57:112-137, 1987.
2. Russo, I.H. and Russo, J. Cancer Surveys, 5:649-670, 1986.
3. Valaoras, V.G., MacMachon, B., Trichopoulus, D. and
   Polychronopoulou, A. Int. J. Cancer 4:350-363, 1969.
4. MacMahon, B. J. Natl. Cancer Inst. 50:21-42, 1973.
5. Krieger, N. J. Natl. Cancer Inst. 30:2-3, 1988.
6. MacMahon, B., Cole, P., Liu, M., Lowe, C.R., Mirra, A.P.,
   Ravinihar, B., Salber, E.J., Valaoras, V.G. and Yuasa, S. Bull.
   WHO 34:209-221, 1970.
7. Yuasa, S. and MacMahon, B. Bull. WHO 42:195-204, 1970.
8. Salber, E.J., Trichopoulos, D. and MacMahon, B. J. Nat. Cancer
   Inst. 43:1013-1024, 1969.
9. Huggins, C.B., Grand, L.C. and Brillantes, F.P. Nature
   189:204-207, 1961.
10. Dao, T.L., Bock, F.G. and Greiner, M.J. J. Natl. Cancer Inst.
    25:991-1003, 1960.
11. Russo, J., Tay, L.K. and Russo, I.H. Breast Cancer Res. Treat
    2:5-73, 1982.
12. Russo, J. Toxicologic Pathol. 11:149-166, 1983.
13. Russo, J., Wilgus, G. and Russo, I.H. Am. J. Pathol.
    96:721-735, 1979.
14. Russo, I.H. and Russo, J. J. Natl. Cancer Inst. 61:1439-1449,
    1978.
15. Russo, J. and Russo, I.H. J. Natl. Cancer Inst. 61:1451-1459,
    1978.
16. Russo, J., Saby, J., Isenberg, W.M. and Russo, I.H. J. Natl.
    Cancer Inst. 59: 435-445, 1977.
17. Russo, I.H., Tewari, M. and Russo, J. In: "Integument and
    Mammary Gland of Laboratory Animals. Jones, T.C., Konishi, Y.,
    Mohr, U. (eds.) Berlin, Springer-Verlag, 1988 (In press).
18. Russo, I.H., Saby, J. and Isenberg, W. Proc. Am. Assoc. Cancer
    Res. 17:463a, 1976.
19. Russo, J., Russo, I.H., van Zwieten, M.J., Robers, A.E. and
    Gusterson, B. In: Integument and Mammary Gland, Monograph
    series on the Pathology of Laboratory Animals. Jones, T.C.,
    Konishi, Y. and Mohr, U. (eds.) Berlin, Springer-Verlag, 1988
    (In Press).
20. Russo, I.H. and Russo, J. Anticancer Res., 8:1247, 1988.
21. Hashimoto, K., Tarnowski, W.M., Lever, W.F. Hautarzt
    18:318-324, 1967.
22. Dvorak, H.F. and Dvorak, A.M. Human Pathol. 3:454-456, 1972.
23. Folkman, J. Cancer Res. 46:467-473, 1986.
24. Kessler, D.A., Langer, R.S., Pless, N.A. and Folkman, J. Int.
    J. Cancer 18:703-709, 1976.
25. Zetter, B.R. Nature (Lond.) 285:41:43, 1980.

26. Azizkhan, R.G., Azizkhan, J.C., Zetter, B.R. and Folkman, J. J. Exp. Med. 152:931-944, 1980.
27. Gospardorowicz, D., Cheng, J., Lui, G.M., Baird, A. and Bohlent, P. Proc. Natl. Acad. Sci. USA 81:6963-6967, 1984.
28. Lobb, R.R. and Fett, J.N. Biochemistry 23:6295-6299, 1984.
29. Lippman, M. Nature 219:33-36, 1968.
30. McBride, W.M. and Bard, J.B.L. J. Exp. Med. 149:507-515, 1979.
31. Ito, I. Anat. Res. 151:489a, 1965.
32. Bekesi, J.G. and Winzler, R.J. J. Biol. Chem. 242:3873-3879, 1967.
33. Bossmann, H.B., Hagopian, A. and Eylar, E.H. Arch. Biochem. Biophys. 130:573-583, 1969.
34. Kraemer, P.M. In: Surfaces of normal and malignant cells. R O. Hynes, ed. Wiley Interscience, New York, pp. 149-198, 1979.
35. Esko, J.D., Rostand, K.S., Weinke, J.L. Science 241:1092-1096, 1988.
36. Codinton, J.F. In: Cellular Membrane and Tumor Cell Behavior. Williams and Wilkins, Baltimore, pp 399-419, 1975.
37. Russo, J., Russo, I.H., Ireland, M. and Saby, J. Proc. Am. Assoc. Cancer Res. 18:149a, 1977.
38. Russo, J., Miller, J. and Russo, I.H. Proc. Am. Assoc. Cancer Res. 23:348a, 1982.
39. Russo, J. and Russo, I.H. IRCS, Med. Sci. 10:877-880, 1982.
40. Russo, J. and Russo, I.H. Am. J. Pathol. 100:497-512, 1980.
41. Russo, I.H., Al-Rayess, M. and Sabharwal, S. Proc. Am. Assoc. Cancer Res. 26:460a, 1985.
42. Russo, I.H., Al-Rayess, M. and Russo, J. Biennial Intl. Breast Cancer Res. Conf. p 87, 1985.
43. Russo, I.H., Pokorzynski, T. and Russo, J. Proc. Am. Assoc. Cancer Res. 27:912a, 1986.
44. Russo, I.H., Frederick, J. and Russo, J. Breast Cancer Res. and Treat. (In Press).
45. Tay, L.K. and Russo, J. Chem. Biol. Interact. 55:13-21, 1985.
46. Ciocca, D.R., Parente, A. and Russo, J. Am. J. Pathol. 109:47-56, 1982.
47. Russo, J. and Russo, I.H. Cancer Res. 40:2671-2687, 1980.
48. Berenblum, I. Cancer Res. 14:471-476, 1954.
49. Frei, J.V. and Harsano, T. Cancer Res. 27:1482-1491, 1967.
50. Kakunaga, T. Cancer Res. 35:1637-1642, 1975.
51. Marquardt, H., Baker, S., Tierney, B., Grover, P.L. and Sims, P. Br. J. Cancer 39:540-547, 1979.
52. Tay, L.K. and Russo, J. J. Natl. Cancer Inst. 67:155-161, 1981.
53. Tay, L.K., and Russo, J. Carcinogenesis 2:1327-1333, 1981.
54. Marchant, J. J. Pathol. Bacteriol. 70:415-418, 1955.
55. Marchant, J. Brit. J. Cancer, 12:55-61, 1958.
56. Russo, J. Russo, I.H., Ireland, M. and Saby, J. Proc. Am. Assoc. Cancer Res. 18:149a, 1977.
57. Hertz, R. In: Chorionic Gonadotropin. Segal, SJ (ed). New York, Plenum Pub Corp, 1980, pp 1-15.
58. Welsch, C.W., Clemens, J.A. and Meites, J. J. Natl. Cancer Inst. 41:465-471, 1968.
59. Grubbs, C.J., Farnell, D.R., Hill, D.L. and McDonough, K.D. J. Natl. Cancer Inst. 74:927-931, 1985.
60. Welsch, C.W. and Meites, J. Cancer 13:601-607, 1969.

61. Rudali, G., Coezy, E. and Chemama, R. J. Natl. Cancer Inst. 49:813-819, 1972.
62. Russo, J., Tay, L.K., Ciocca, D.R. and Russo, I.H. Environ. Health Perspect 49:185-199, 1983.
63. Henderson, B.E., Koss, R.K., Judd, H.L., Krailo, M.D. and Pike, M.C. Cancer 56:1206-1208, 1985.
64. Pike, M.C., Henderson, B.E. and Krailo, M.D. Lancet II:926-930, 1983.
65. Welsch, C.W., Goodrich-Smith, M., Brown, C.K. and Roth, L. Breast Cancer Res. Treat. 1:225-232, 1981.
66. Daniel, C.W., Silberstein, G.B. and Strickland, P. Cancer Res. 47:6052-6057, 1987.
67. Freeman, C.S. and Topper, Y.J. J. Toxicol. Environ. Health 4:269-282, 1978.
68. Fechner, R.E. Cancer 39: 2764-2771, 1977.
69. Stern, E. and Mickey, M.R. Brit. J. Cancer 23:391-400, 1969.
70. Garza-Flores, J., Cravioto, M.C., Del Real Mora, O., Anderson, J., Landeros, J., Diaz Sanchez, V., Lichtenberg, R. and Perez-Palacios, G. Medico Interamericano 4:66-71, 1985.
71. Kledizk, B.S., Bradle, C.J. and Meites, J. Cancer Res. 34:2953-2956, 1974.
72. Kahn, R.A. and Baker, B.L. Endocrinol 75:818-821, 1964.
73. Edgren, R.A. In: Contraception: The chemical Control of Fertility. Ednicer, DL (ed.), New York, Marcel Dekker, Inc. 1969 pp 23-68.
74. Calaf, G., Russo, I.H., Roi, L.D. and Russo, J. In Vitro Cell Develop. Biol. 22:135-140, 1986.
75. McManus, M.J. and Welsch, C.W. Cancer Res. 41:3300-3305, 1981.
76. Russo, J. and Russo, I.H. Am. J. Pathol., 100:497-512, 1980.
77. Minasian-Batmanian, L.C. and Jabara, A.G. Br. J. Cancer 43:832-841, 1981.
78. Rose, D.P. and Noonan, J.J. Cancer Res. 42:35-38, 1982.
79. Livolsi, V.A., Stadel, B.V., Kelsey, J.L., Holford, T.R. and White, C. New Engl. J. Med. 299:381-385, 1978.
80. Pastides, H., Kelsey, J.L., Livolsi, V.A., Holford, T.R., Fischer, D.B. and Goldenberg, I.S. J. Natl. Cancer Inst. 71:5-9, 1983.
81. Cole, P.T. Cancer 39:1906-1918, 1977.
82. Cancer and Steroid Hormone Study of the Centers for Disease Control and the National Institute of Child Health and Human Development. N. Engl. J. Med. 315:405-411, 1986.
83. Wang, D.Y. and Fentiman, I.S. Breast Cancer Res. Treat. 6:5-36, 1985.
84. McCann, J. Oncol. Times VII:35, 1985.
85. WHO Collaborative Study of Neoplasia and Steroid Contraceptives. Lancet II:1207-1208, 1984.
86. Vessey, M.P., Doll, R., Jones, K., McPherson, K., and Yeates, D. Br. Med. J. 1:1757-1760, 1979.
87. Thomas, D.B. Cancer Res. 38:3991-4000, 1978.
88. Rosner, D. and Lane, W.W. Cancer 57:591-596, 1986.
89. Concannon, P., Altszuler, N., Hampshire, J., Butler, R. and Hansel, W. Endocrinol. 106:1173-1177, 1980.

90. Fowler, E.H., Vaughn, T., Gotcsik, F., Reichart, P. and Reed, C. In: Pharmacology of Steroid Contraceptive Drugs, Garattini S and Berendes HW (eds.) New York, Raven Press, 1977, pp 185-210.
91. Frank, D.W., Kirton, K.T., Murchison, T.E., Quinlan, J.W., Coleman, M.E., Gilbertson, T.J., Feenstra, E.S. and Kimball, M.A. Fertil. Steril. 31:340-346, 1979.
92. Lanari, C., Molinolo, A.A. and Pasqualini, C.D. J. Natl. Cancer Inst. 77:157-164, 1986.
93. Lanari, C., Molinolo, A.A. and Pasqualini, C.D. Cancer Letters 33:215-223, 1986.
94. MacLaughlin, D.T. and Richardson, G.S. J. Steroid Biochem. 10:371-377, 1979.
95. Huggins, C., Moon, R. and Morii, S. Proc. Natl. Acad. Sci. 48:379-386, 1979.
96. Jabara, A.G. Br. J. Cancer 21:418-429, 1967.
97. Kelly, P.A., Asseline, J., Labrie, F., Raynaud, J.P. In: Progress in Cancer Research and Therapy, McGuire WL, Raynaud JP, Baulieu EE (eds) New York, Raven Press, 1977, pp 85-102.
98. Wang, D.Y. and Fentimen, I.S. Breast Cancer Res. Treat. 6:5-36, 1985.
99. Vessey, M.P., McPherson, K., Roberts, M.M., Neil, A. and Jones, L. Br. J. Cancer 52:625-628, 1985.
100. England, P.C., Skinner, L.G., Cottrell, K.M. and Sellwood, R.A. Br. J. Cancer 30:571-576, 1974.
101. Henderson, B.E., Berkins, V., Rosario, I., Casagrande, J. and Pike, M.C. N. Engl. J. Med. 293:790-795, 1975.
102. Trichopoulos, D., Brown, J.B., Garas, J., Papionnaou, A. and Macmahon, B. J. Natl. Cancer Inst. 57:603-608, 1981.
103. Richardson, G.S. and McLaughlin, D.H. UICC Technical Report, 565, 1978.
104. Pike, M.C., Henderson, B.E., Casagrande, J.T., Rosario, I. and Grey, G.E. Br. J. Cancer 43:72-76, 1981.
105. Pike, M.C., Henderson, B.E., Krailo, M.D., Duke, A. and Roy, S. Lancet II:926-930, 1983.
106. Rosner, D. and Lane, W.W. Cancer 57:591-596, 1986.
107. Thomas, D.B. Cancer Res. 38:3991-4000, 1978.
108. Vessey, M.P., Doll, R., Jones, K., McPherson, K. and Yeates, D. Br. Med. J. 1:1757-1760, 1979.

13

STEROID RECEPTORS AND BREAST CANCER: CURRENT STATUS AND NEW APPLICATIONS FOR RECEPTOR-DIRECTED DIAGNOSIS AND THERAPY

E.R. DeSOMBRE, A. HUGHES, W.J. KING, S.J. GATLEY, J.L. SCHWARTZ AND P.V. HARPER

Ben May Institute, Departments of Radiology and Radiation Oncology, The University of Chicago, 5841 S. Maryland Avenue, Chicago, IL 60637

INTRODUCTION

There is a long history for the clinical use of the hormone dependence of human breast cancer. In the last several decades our increased knowledge of the basic mechanisms involved in this hormone dependence have led to improvements in the diagnosis, treatment and follow-up of breast cancer patients. With the incidence of breast cancer at more than 120,000 new cases per year in the United States, leading to over 40,000 deaths due to this disease, it is clear that there is still a major need for new approaches which can reduce the incidence and mortality of this disease. For some of these improvements, knowledge of, and intervention based upon, the presence of steroid receptors in lesions of the breast can be a key to decreased mortality. This chapter will summarize the earlier advances based on endocrine approaches to the diagnosis and therapy of breast cancer and discuss current developments which can lead to reduced incidence, improved diagnosis, and more effective therapy based on the presence of steroid receptors in these lesions.

HORMONE DEPENDENCE OF BREAST CANCER

Over 150 years ago Cooper had observed a relationship between ovarian secretions and the growth of human breast cancer (1). The first clinical application of this relationship was the report in 1896 by Beatson that several premenopausal breast cancer patients on whom he performed oophorectomy experienced remission of widespread disease (2). However, a major impetus for the use of endocrine ablative surgery for advanced breast cancer followed the report in 1952 by Huggins and Bergenstal (3) that in postmenopausal patients with metastatic breast cancer adrenalectomy could effect striking remission of disease. Not long afterward reports from the U.S (4) and Sweden (5) showed that hypophysectomy could likewise bring about remission of metastatic breast cancer. Hormone additive therapy was studied during the 1940s, using large amounts of estrogens (6) or androgens (7), and was also found to be effective in some metastatic breast cancer patients. All these studies, however, indicated that while endocrine therapies could be effective in those patients who responded, fewer than 1/3 of all patients received objective benefit. It was therefore important to establish methods which could *a priori* identify breast cancer patients who were likely to respond.

<u>Estrogen Receptor Assays</u>

The basis for the development of such methods were observations that the normal hormone-dependent tissues of the reproductive tract of experimental animals were able to concentrate administered estrogens, while non-target tissues for estrogens lacked this capacity (8). Even using a very simple in vitro assay to measure the specific uptake of ^{3}H-labeled estradiol by slices of breast cancer we were able to identify the group of patients who were likely to respond to endocrine ablative therapy (9). As is now well known, the capability to take up and retain estrogens relates to the substantial concentrations of estrogen receptor (ER) protein in these target tissues. As this was appreciated more convenient assays, not requiring fresh tissue, were designed, first using sedimentation analysis (10), then titration analysis (11) of ^{3}H-E2 binding in extracts of the breast cancers. As these methods came into more common use at many major medical centers throughout the world it was possible to assess their usefulness to predict response to endocrine therapies.

CURRENT STATUS OF STEROID RECEPTORS IN BREAST CANCER
<u>Clinical Correlations with Steroid Receptors</u>

Already by 1974, at the meeting held by the Breast Cancer Task Force of the National Cancer Institute (NCI), it was apparent that with few exceptions the patients who responded to endocrine therapies were those whose cancers contained ER (12). However, not all patients whose cancers contained ER benefited from endocrine therapies. Considerable effort was expended to fine tune the assay or establish additional criteria to more accurately identify those patients who responded. When the NCI subsequently convened a consensus development meeting (13) to assess the usefulness of steroid receptors in breast cancer much more data was available. Results from nearly 2,000 patient trials clearly indicated that few remissions were seen in patients whose cancers lacked ER, while about 55% of ER+ patients had objective remissions to various endocrine therapies (14,15). Even though clinicians had developed certain clinical criteria, which some felt helped identify patients likely to benefit from endocrine therapy, a study of various factors indicated that ER was in fact the most important parameter for predicting response (16). Furthermore, it was found that consideration of the quantity of ER (17,18) could improve the identification of patients most likely to respond.

Another approach was suggested by Horwitz and McGuire(19). Following up on basic studies which indicated that in estrogen target tissues the synthesis of progestin receptors (PgR) constitutes a response to estrogen, they suggested that information on the presence of PgR as well as ER in the lesions might be better correlated with response (20). Indeed, subsequent reports clearly indicate that patients with lesions containing both receptors are more likely to respond to endocrine therapies, than those with only one of these receptors (summarized in 15).

As ER and PgR were more commonly assayed in excised breast cancers, other useful clinical information emerged. In particular, it became clear that patients with receptor positive lesions had a more favorable prognosis than did patients with receptor negative cancers (21-23). It appears that in general the disease-free survival of ER+ and PgR+ stage 1 and 2 breast cancer patients is longer than that of their receptor negative counterparts. While other factors, such as menopausal status and lymph node involvement, are also important, the steroid receptor status appears to be an independent prognostic factor. It also appears that patients with receptor positive lesions have a longer survival, but this may in part be due to their response to endocrine therapies. Since the Consensus Meeting it has been commonly accepted practice to routinely assay all human breast cancers for ER and PgR, and in clinical studies the receptor status is often used to stratify patients for treatment.

Newer Assays for ER and PgR

Even though clinically useful information has resulted from conventional titration assays for ER and PgR, performed on extracts of surgically excised breast cancers, these assays are not without problems. There has been difficulty reproducing such assay results among different laboratories and considerable effort has gone into establishing protocols and quality assurance procedures to insure that there is a reasonable degree of reproducibility of results from one laboratory to another. The steroid receptors are quite labile proteins, and are generally even more unstable in homogenates of cancer tissue. In addition, there has been considerable interest in studying the heterogeneity of expression of ER in the cancers. Obviously, homogenization of the lesion precludes assessment of heterogeneity of ER in that tissue. Equally serious, since one can not carry out a histopathologic characterization of the tissue actually being homogenized, it is not possible to know which cells contain ER.

With antibodies to ER newer assays for the receptor, not dependent on the binding of steroid to the receptor protein, could be developed. However, the prerequisite purification of ER was a challenge because of its lability and the minute concentration of this protein in tissues. ER was eventually purified and anti-ER antibodies were produced, first with ER purified from calf uterus (24), and then also from ER of the MCF-7 breast cancer cell line (25). With a library of monoclonal antibodies specific for ER, both an enzyme immunoassay (ER-EIA), based on bead technology, and a immunocytochemical assay (ER-ICA) were developed and tested. The ER-EIA results have been found to correlate very well with results of conventional biochemical titration assays (26,27) and are simpler to perform with good quality

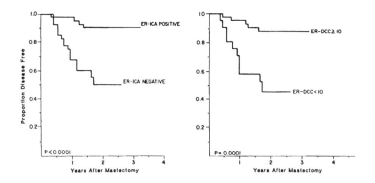

Fig.1. Disease-free interval as related to ER-ICA status (left) and ER-DCC status (right). Patients were postmenopausal breast cancer patients at high risk of recurrence, entered into the Danish Breast Cancer Cooperative Group adjuvant therapy trials. ER assays were performed independently on the primary lesions. ER-DCC groups divided at 10 fmole/mg protein. From reference 31.

control. This assay procedure has now been approved for diagnostic use in the U.S. and is available in kit form.

The ER-ICA procedure allows assessment of tissue and subcellular localization of ER. Initial studies clearly indicated that ER is a nuclear protein (28), despite the fact that it is readily extracted from cells with buffers of low ionic strength. Other results, both biochemical (29) and autoradiographic (30), confirmed the nuclear localization of ER. When we evaluated the immunostaining for ER in sections of human breast cancers, which were also assayed for ER by conventional steroid binding assays, the two methods showed general agreement. Initially we made a simple assessment based on whether the sections were predominantly stained for nuclear ER, or not. With such a simple classification the prognostic utility of the ER-ICA result was found to be similar to that of conventional assays, in a collaborative study with the Danish Breast Cancer Group (31), Fig. 1. Furthermore, in this patient population the ER-ICA status appeared to be a prognostic factor independent from the lymph node status, Fig. 2A. While patients with ER-ICA negative lesions and more than 4 positive lymph nodes had the shortest disease free interval (DFI) as expected, patients with more than 4 positive nodes but ER-ICA+ cancers had a better prognosis and a DFI similar to patients with fewer positive lymph nodes but lacking substantial ER as indicated by ER-ICA. In fact, when evaluated for length of survival the ER-ICA status appeared to be a stronger prognostic indicator than the lymph node status, but this may relate to the randomization of some of the patients to adjuvant antiestrogen therapy (31).

Immunohistochemical studies of the heterogeneity of expression of ER and PgR in human breast cancer suggest that this parameter may be of considerable utility. The impor-

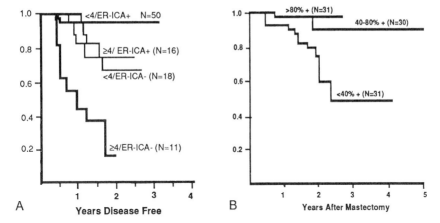

Fig. 2. ER-ICA and Lymph Node Status Related to Disease-free Survival and % ER-ICA Positive Cells Related to Overall Survival. Follow-up data was obtained from the postmeno-pausal breast cancer patients in the adjuvant therapy trials of the Danish Breast Cancer Group described in Fig. 1. A (left) Proportion of patients disease free versus time after mastectomy is plotted for the patients according to the lymph node status (<4 or ≥4 lymph nodes involved) and the ER-ICA status of the cancer. B (right) Proportion of patients living versus time after mastectomy is plotted according to the proportion of cancer cells which stained positively for nuclear ER by the ER-ICA procedure. Numbers in parenthesis correspond to the number of patients in each group. From reference 31.

tance of being able to assess the cellular localization of steroid receptors is especially clear when the excised lesion contains mixed cell types. For example, we have seen some samples, found to be a low ER+ by conventional steroid binding assays, where the only cells stained for ER were normal or hyperplastic epithelia adjacent to the cancer. In one of these a subsequently assayed lymph node metastasis showed no ER by ER-ICA or steroid binding assays. It is therefore likely that some of the tissue samples with low ER content may be ER positive by conventional ER assays due to their content of normal or benign epithelium which contain ER, while the cancer itself lacks ER. Such false positive assays can be avoided by using immunohistochemical assays to identify the cells containing the receptor.

ER-ICA assays have also shown that the expression of ER is frequently heterogeneous in the breast cancers themselves. The clinical or biological implications of this heterogeneity are not yet clear, but could be of substantial relevance to the clinical course and treatment response. In the Danish study (31), it was apparent that there was a significantly different prognosis for lesions with differing proportions of ER-ICA positive cancer cells. When patient prognosis was compared with the percent ER positive cells in the breast cancers, significant differences were associated with lesions with 40% or greater as opposed to < 40% ER positive cells (Fig. 2B), while there was no significant difference between patients with 40-80%

and > 80% ER-ICA positive cells. One explanation for this result is that the ER-containing cells are controlling the overall biology and response of the lesion, such as by a paracrine mechanism. There is some evidence for such a mechanism in that breast cancer cells appear to produce growth factors in response to estrogen treatment (32). Such a paracrine mechanism would explain why one sees remissions of cancers which may contain a significant proportion of ER negative cells. This would imply that growth of the cells lacking ER may depend on estrogen-induced growth factors produced by the ER positive cells. It will be important to obtain more extensive correlations of ER distribution in breast cancers with clinical performance and responses to endocrine therapies to appreciate the relevence of the heterogeneity of ER distribution.

Available information on the expression of ER in the normal breast has been somewhat controversial. Conventional ER assays have shown either very low values for ER in the normal human breast and in some cases no significant ER could be detected. The tissues generally assayed to provide the available data consisted of samples from reductive mammoplasty or apparently normal breast tissue adjacent to a lesion in a mastectomy sample. It is clear that in such samples the proportion of normal breast epithelium is very small, so that the assay of extracts from an homogenate of such samples would mainly reflect the extraneous tissue. With Josef Tóth, we used ER-ICA to assess ER in such apparently normal breast epithelium (33). Our results indicate that there is heterogeneity in the expression of ER in the normal breast epithelium. Staining was seen in extralobular and intralobular terminal ducts as well as in the terminal ductules. There was a significant range in stain intensity as well as in the proportion of stained cells. The staining was restricted to the epithelial elements. These ER-ICA results are consistent with the low ER values generally obtained with steroid binding assays since the epithelium constitutes a very small proportion of most such samples. Preliminary results (33) of ER-ICA studies of hyperplastic epithelia in the breast have shown more uniform staining than was evident in the normal breast. However, we need to know the effect of the menstual cycle on the expression of ER in the normal and hyperplastic breast epithelium before we can interpret differences in ER in these tissues. Nonetheless, immunohistochemical studies of ER have the potential to clarify our understanding of the expression of ER in the normal breast epithelium and highlight clinically important differences in ER of the normal, hyperplastic and neoplastic breast epithelium.

NEW APPLICATIONS OF STEROID RECEPTORS

Despite the advances in diagnosis of steroid receptor positive lesions and the increased use of endocrine therapy for treatment of such breast cancer patients, at best only 25-30% overall of metastatic breast cancer patients will respond to endocrine therapies. Indeed most metastatic breast cancer patients will eventually die from their disease. To reduce the mortality due to breast cancer our greatest opportunities are to reduce the incidence of breast cancer, to obtain earlier detection and more definitive diagnosis when the disease can be most effectively treated, and to develop more effective therapies for patients who develop metastatic disease. While these are quite general goals, creative application of knowledge of steroid receptors can help create new opportunities to reach these goals.

Early Intervention

There is a general belief that most, if not all, breast cancers arise in a hormone dependent state and that in the course of the disease, the normal hormonal constraints are circumvented, giving rise to increased hormone autonomy. This autonomy may arise concomitant with loss of expression of ER, since ER would no longer be necessary to the growth control of the cells, or along with continued expression of ER, even though the presence of ER would then be superfluous to growth control. However, if a high proportion of the early lesions are hormone dependent it should be possible to use hormonal intervention to treat them more effectively. Considering that there is evidence that certain proliferative benign lesions of the breast are associated with a significantly higher risk of breast cancer, it will be important to assess the potential hormone dependence of such lesions. While the biologic dependence on estrogen may be difficult to establish in patients, the content and distribution of ER are more readily studied. Our preliminary results suggest that proliferative hyperplasias of the breast show more uniform ER expression than do carcinomas in situ or invasive breast cancers (33). If this can be confirmed and extended it would suggest that more agressive and extensive hormonal intervention should be attempted in patients with such high risk lesions. In fact, the prophylactic use of antiestrogens has been suggested without such biologic data because of the potential benefit of such intervention. Since the long term effects of treatment with antiestrogens, which are partial estrogen agonists, are not clear at the present, other apporaches should be considered as well. Another alternative, which has been successfully used for endometrial hyperplasias, is treatment with progestins. The ability of progestins to antagonize estrogen proliferative effects and possibly effect terminal differentiation of hyperplastic epithelia could benefit patients with premalignant proliferative lesions of the breast as well. What is essential at this time is to make use of the tools, ie. immunohistochemical assays for ER and PgR, to obtain more extensive data on the steroid receptor distribution in various benign lesions of the breast to correlate with the biologic potential of these lesions.

Early diagnosis and detection of ER & PgR positive lesions

One of the significant changes evident over the last several decades is the earlier detection of breast cancers. This is probably relates to increased frequency of breast self examination and the more general use of routine mammographic screening. Some lesions, not evident on physical examination, are being found by followup of suspicious mammograms. Increasingly needle aspiration biopsies are being used to diagnose suspected lesions using radiographic needle localization based on the mammograms. With the ability to assess ER or PgR by ICA on cell smears, it is now possible to determine the probable steroid receptor status in the limited amounts of material from such biopsies as well as from excisional biopsies of minimal lesions at the time of histologic diagnosis. Although the use of a relatively benign adjuvant treatment with antiestrogens might be considered without steroid receptor results, such data is essential to obtain a complete understanding of the clinical results and to make the most effective use of therapy trials of early intervention.

There is also a potential for systemic detection of steroid receptor positive lesions using suitable steroid receptor-directed radioligands. The last few years have seen substantial improvements in the synthetic chemistry of the positron emitting, ^{18}F ligands in general, and have led to initial optimism about the use of positron emission tomography (PET) scanning for steroid receptor containing lesions (34). The improved signal to noise ratio and 3 dimensional accuracy associated with PET scanning has considerable attraction for detection of breast cancers.

Even with more conventional radiologic imaging methods there are some indications that detection of distant ER+ lesions may be possible. With the development of the halodestannylation reaction (35) it is now possible to obtain high yields of radioiodine-labeled steroids very rapidly, as required for preparation of ligands containing nuclides of short half lives. Furthermore with the commercial availability of virtually pure iodine-123, a 13.2 hr half-life nuclide which emits a 159 keV γ–ray, conventional nuclear or SPECT (Single Photon Emission Computed Tomography) imaging can be used with [^{123}I]iodoestrogens to image ER+ breast cancers. Promising preliminary images of ER+ breast cancers have been reported using 16α[^{123}I] iodoestradiol (36). Possibly improved iodoestrogens, containing the more stable vinyl iodine-carbon bond, have the potential to improve the stability of the iodoestrogens in vivo. We are currently investigating the use of a non-steroidal, triphenylethylene-based iodovinyl estrogen (37) and others have begun studies with 17α–iodovinyl-11β–methoxyestradiol (38).

<u>Estrogen receptor-directed therapy</u>

While the endocrine-induced remissions of metastatic breast cancer are important, and clearly increase the survival of patients who respond, there are in fact few cures. Patients die of distant disease as much as 10-20 years after remission to hormone therapy. This may follow from the fact that current endocrine therapies are cytostatic, not cytotoxic, ie. they inhibit cell growth but do not kill the cancer cells. Endocrine ablation removes the source of estrogen (oophorectomy) or androgen which is peripherally converted to estrogen (adrenalectomy). Aromatase inhibitors prevent, or reduce the rate of, conversion of androgens to estrogens. Antiestrogens probably compete with endogenous estrogens at the receptor, at least in part thereby inhibiting the estrogenic action. However, with each of these therapies the estrogen-dependent cancer cells may remain dormant for a long time. Hence, if the precarious endocrine balance is disturbed, as with compensatory production of estrogen, these cancer cells could begin to proliferate and disseminate. Indications that patients appeared to relapse once short term tamoxifen adjuvant therapy was stopped has led to trials of long term (5 years) or indefinite continuation of such therapy in the hope of improved disease free survival. Furthermore, even though their growth is suppressed, some of the surviving cells could undergo mutations to circumvent the hormonal dependent constraints resulting in a tumor that can grow under estrogen suppressive conditions.

Thus, there is some attraction to the concept of a cytotoxic endocrine therapy. We believe that the estrogen receptor can be the basis for such an approach. One of the unique characteristics of the estrogen receptor is that it is a nuclear protein which, when associated with estrogen, binds tightly to distinct steroid response elements in the DNA . This characteristic could be useful for receptor-directed therapy. Our approach is to synthesize an Auger electron emitting, estrogen receptor-directed ligand as a means of bringing the short range, highly potent Auger electron cascade into the vicinity of the DNA where it can cause irreparable damage. Unlike β decay which is the expulsion of a single electron from the nucleus of the decaying atom, Auger electron decay results in a "shower" of low energy electrons. As illustrated in Fig. 3 for the 4.4 hr half life nuclide bromine-80m, the process is started by emission of a k-shell conversion electron. This inner shell vacancy is filled by an electron from a higher energy level, resulting in a high energy state which leads to the emission of either a photon or another valence electron. The energy of the emitted Auger electron corresponds to the energy difference between the initial and final states of the electron which changed levels, minus the binding energy of the emitted electron. The process of filling the initial vacancy therefore not only results in the emission of an electron, but the creation of another valence shell vacancy. As the process continues and moves to the outer shells, a greater number of electrons are emitted, in effect a shower of electrons, the number and energy distribution of which is characteristic of the atom involved. For bromine-80m, illustrated in Fig. 3, the Auger process results in the emission of an average of 8 electrons in the condensed state (39).

What is biologically important is that the energy of these emitted Auger electrons is very low, typically under 10 keV, and hence their range is only nanometers. This results in highly concentrated radiation near the site of decay. Evidence from studies of the Auger electron emission of the nuclide, I-125, when incorporated into DNA have shown that such radiation is very effective in killing cells (40). In fact, the theoretical possibility to use this ap-

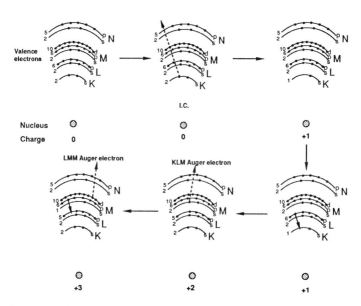

Fig. 3. Representation of an Auger decay scheme of bromine-80m. The decay is initiated by internal conversion, represented as the emission of a K-shell electron (middle top), resulting in a +1 charge on the atom (top right). The subsequent filling of the K-shell vacancy (bottom right) results in the emission of a KLM Auger electron (ie. M electron emitted following the L to K shell transition), giving an atom with a +2 charge (middle bottom). The cascade continues, as represented by an M to L shell transition and emission of an LMM Auger electron (bottom left).

proach was described in studies in tissue culture, with [125I] 16α–iodoestradiol (41). However, since iodine-125 has a half-life of 60 days, it was necessary to freeze down the iodoestradiol-loaded cells for months to accumulate sufficient decays to demonstrate the radiotoxicity. Oviously an Auger electron emitting nuclide of considerably shorter half life is needed to be useful in vivo.

One attraction of bromine-80m is that it's 4.4 hr half life is similar to the biological half life of ER (42). Thus if one can load an estrogen receptor with this nuclide bound to an appropriate ligand there is a good likelihood that the nuclide would decay while still bound to the receptor at the DNA. To demonstrate that this approach is feasible it was necessary to determine how many bromine-80m decays are required to kill a cell. Clearly there are a limited number (ie. 500-10,000) of ER molecules per cell in breast cancers so fewer than 1,000 decays per cell must show radiotoxic activity. It was also necessary to design, synthesize and test a bromine-containing ER binding ligand to demonstrate that the addition of bromine to an estrogen was compatible with retention of its high binding affinity for the receptor. The proposed bromoestrogen must be specifically taken up by ER target tissues in vivo, and be able to kill ER+ cells in vitro and vivo. Finally, the radioligand should have only minimal side effects in vivo, compatible with its use in patients.

Because of its short half life we produce the bromine-80m locally in our CS-15 cyclotron using a (p,n) reaction with a selenium-80 target. Initially we prepared bromine-80m labeled bromodeoxyuridine, [80mBr] BrUdR, to establish the radiotoxic potential of this nuclide when actually incorporated in DNA. When incubated for 18 hr with MCF-7 cells [80mBr] BrUdR which was incorporated into DNA killed the cells, but the same nuclide present in the medium as bromide ion, or more uniformly distributed in the cells (bromoantipyrine) had little lethal effect (43). This not only showed that bromine-80m could kill cells, but importantly, that nuclear localization was necessary for its radiotoxicity.

With the long doubling time of MCF-7 cells (about 36 hr) and the short half life of bromine-80m estimates of mean lethal dose are complicated in studies where the incubation time is long compared to the half life of the nuclide. Therefore, we studied Chinese Hamster Ovary (CHO) cells which have a doubling time of 16 hr. In these studies we used a 2 hr incubation with [80mBr] BrUdR to be able to quantify the incorporation of the short half life nuclide. The survival curve, Fig. 4, had an initial plateau at about 75% survival which was compatible

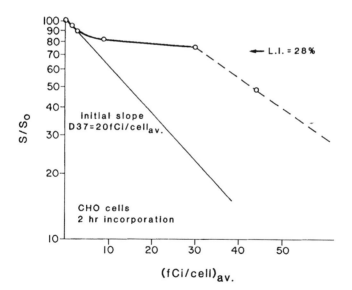

Fig. 4. Survival curve of CHO cells treated with [80mBr] BrUdR for 2 hr. After 2 hr some of the plated cells were washed, homogenized and TCA precipitated to establish incorporation of radionuclide, and others, washed and given fresh control media for growth and colony assay after one week. Labeling index was determined from autoradiograms of cells plated and incubated with [80mBr] BrUdR for 2 hr on glass slides and exposed to emulsion for one day.

with the 28% labeling index found by autoradiography. Extrapolation of the initial slope gave a mean lethal dose of about 20 fCi/cell (average) which, when corrected for the labeling index, corresponded to about 50 molecules per cell. Subsequent studies with synchronized CHO cells (43), with a 75% labeling index in a 2 hr incubation with [80mBr] BrUdR, showed a mean lethal dose of 43 atoms of bromine-80m per cell. These results are encouraging in that they indicate that the numbers of atoms of bromine-80m incorporated in DNA needed for killing cells are lower than the numbers of ER present in ER+ cancers. Hence, ER-directed therapy with bromine-80m-labeled estrogens appears feasible, assuming that there is not an appreciable reduction in lethality of the decays of the nuclide associated with or incorporated into DNA.

Recently we have been studying a number of bromoestrogens, both steroidal and based on the triphenylethylene structure (37) to determine an appropriate bromine-80m-labeled estrogen receptor ligand to use for the attempted radiotherapy. The non-steroidal estrogen, 2-[80mBr]bromo-1,1-bis(4-hydroxyphenyl)-1-phenylethylene, [80mBr]Br-BHPE, was prepared by the halodestannylation reaction (44), and found to bind to the estrogen receptor, Fig. 5. Comparing the decay corrected 2.68 x 10⁶ DPM of [80mBr]Br-BHPE bound to ER on sedimentation analysis with the 1.26 x 10⁴ DPM for [³H] estradiol, the specific activity for this preparation of [80mBr]Br-BHPE was found to be 8700 Ci/mmole. As is seen in Fig. 5 the binding to ER was specific since it was inhibited by unlabeled DES. Furthermore, we have

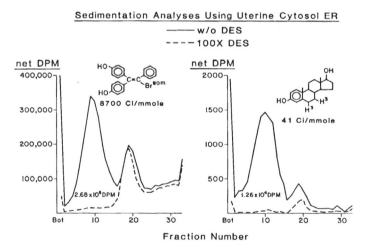

Fig. 5. Sedimentation analysis of the binding of [80mBr]Br-BHPE to low salt extractable ER from immature rat uterus. Saturating concentrations of [³H]E2 or [80mBr]Br-BHPE alone (solid line) or along with 1 µmolar DES (dashed line) were incubated with ER, excess estrogens removed with DCC and the labeled extracts analyzed on 10-30% sucrose gradients in low salt buffer. From reference 44.

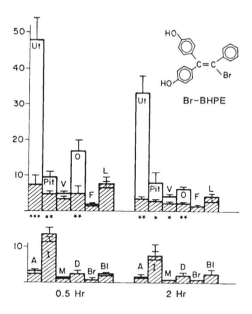

Fig. 6. Specific uptake of [80mBr]Br-BHPE in tissues of the immature female rat. The [80mBr]Br-BHPE was administered i.p., alone (open bars) or with 1 µg DES (crosshatched bars) and at each time point 3 animals from each group were sacrificed, the indicated tissues were excised, blotted, weighed wet, and assayed for radioactivity. Results are presented as mean % of injected dose per gram wet weight of tissue. Error bars indicate S.D. of the mean. Tissue codes are: uterus (Ut); pituitary (Pit); vagina (V); ovary (O); fat (F); liver (L); adrenal (A); intestine (I); leg muscle (M); hemidiaphragm (D); brain (Br); and blood (Bl). Statistical significance of concentrations in each tissue comparing the tissue from animals without and with concomitant DES administration: *, P<0.05; **, P<0.02; ***, P<0.002. From reference 44.

also shown that specific anti-ER antibodies recognize the complex with [80mBr]Br-BHPE, additional evidence of its binding to the receptor (44).

Is [80mBr]Br-BHPE taken up by ER+ tissue in vivo? Studies thus far are also encouraging, Fig. 6. The [80mBr]Br-BHPE was administrated alone or along with 1 µg DES to immature rats and the radioactivity present in various tissues at 0.5 and 2 hr was determined. Specific, ie. DES inhibitable, uptake was found for ER+ target tissues of the rat at both 0.5 and 2 hr. Most other tissues showed low levels of radioactivity. Tissues involved in the excretion of the estrogen, such as the liver and intestine, while showing appreciable radioactivity, did not show a reduction of radioactivity when DES was coadministered. Since only the nuclear Auger electron decays should be radiotoxic, the sometimes significant non-specific levels of bromine-80m in non-target tissues, which are not inhibited by DES and thus are probably not nuclear, should not be radiotoxic. The validity of this assumption will be tested as we are able to prepare bromine-80m-labeled estrogens at the higher specific activities needed to test its radiotoxicity. At that time we should also be able to assess any side effects due to the 17 min half life, β–emitting daughter, bromine-80. With new target design and dry distillation recovery, thereby avoiding dilution of the specific activity by halogens present in solvents, we expect to be able to produce >100 mCi quantities of bromine-80m for testing. Finally, since iodine-123 produces Auger electrons in addition to its diagnostically useful 159 keV γ-ray, it is possible that different doses of the same iodine-123-labeled iodoestrogen could be used for imaging, to determine whether ER is present in a lesion, and then for treatment.

ACKNOWLEDGEMENTS

These investigations were supported by the National Institutes of Health (Grants CB 43969, CB 14358, CA 14599, CA 27476, HD 15513), The American Cancer Society, Abbott Laboratories, The Women's Board of the Cancer Research Foundation, and The Jules J. Reingold Fellowship Fund.

REFERENCES
1. Cooper, A.P. In: The Principles and Practice of Surgery, vol 1, E. Cox, London, 1836, pp. 333-335.
2. Beatson, G.T. Lancet 2: 104-107, 1896.
3. Huggins, C., and Bergenstal, D.M. Cancer Res. 12: 134-141,1952.
4. Pearson, O.H., Roy, B.S., and Harrold, C.C. J. Am. Med. Assoc.161: 17-21, 1956.
5. Luft, R. and Olivecrona,
6. Haddow, A., Watkinson, J.M., and Spinelli, J.J. Br. Med. J. 2: 393-398, 1944.
7. Nathanson, I.T. Cancer 5: 754-762, 1952.
8. Jensen, E.V., and Jacobson, H.I. Rec. Prog. Horm. Res. 18: 387-414, 1962.
9. Jensen, E.V., Block, G.E., Smith, S., Kyser, K. and DeSombre, E.R. Natl. Cancer Inst. Monogr. 34: 55-70, 1971.
10. Jensen, E.V., Smith, S., and DeSombre, E.R. J. Steroid Biochem. 7: 905-916, 1976.
11. Rodbard, D., Munson, P.J., and Thakur A.K. Cancer 46: 2907-2918, 1980.
12. McGuire, W.L., Carbone, P.P., and Vollmer, E.P. (editors) Estrogen Receptors in Human Breast Cancer, Raven Press, New York, 1975.
13. DeSombre, E.R., Carbone, P.P., Jensen, E.V., McGuire, W.L., Wells, S.A., Wittliff, J.L., and Lipsett, M.B. New Engl. J. Med. 301: 1011-1012, 1979.
14. Cancer (Suppl) 46: 2759-2964 , 1980.
15. DeSombre, E.R. In: The Breast, (eds R.W. McDivitt, H.A. Oberman, L. Ozzello, N. Kaufman) Williams and Wilkins Publishers, Baltimore, 1984, pp. 149-174.
16. Byar, D.P., Sears, M.E., and McGuire, W.L. Europ. J. Cancer 15: 299-310, 1979.
17. DeSombre, E.R. and Jensen, E.V. Cancer 46: 2783-2788, 1980.
18. Paridaens, R., Sylvester, R.J., Ferrazzi, E., Legros, N., Leclercq. G., and Heuson, J.C. Cancer 46: 2889-2895, 1980.
19. Horwitz, K.G. and McGuire, W.L. Steroids 25: 497-502, 1975.
20. Horwitz, K.B., McGuire, W.L., Pearson, O.H., and Segaloff, A. Science 189: 726-727, 1975.
21. Knight, W.A., Livingston, R.B., Gregory, E.J. and McGuire, W.L. Cancer Res. 37: 4669-4671, 1977.

22. Rich, M.A., Furmanski, P., and Brooks, S.C. Cancer Res. 38: 4292-4298, 1978.
23. Maynard, P.W., Bishop, R.W., Elston, C.W., Haybittle, J.L., and Griffiths, K. Cancer Res. 38: 4292-4295, 1978.
24. Greene, G.L., Closs, L.E., Fleming, H., DeSombre, E.R., and Jensen, E.V. Proc. Natl. Acad. Sci. USA 74: 3681-3685, 1977.
25. Greene, G.L., Nolan, C., Engler, J.P., and Jensen, E.V. Proc. Natl. Acad. Sci. USA 77: 5115-5119, 1980.
26. Leclercq, G., Bojar, H., Goussard, J., Nicholson, R.I., Pichon, M-F., Piffanelli, A., Pousette, A., Thorpe, S., and Lonsdorfer, M. Cancer Res. 46: 4233s-4236s, 1986.
27. Jordan, V.C., Jacobson, H.I., and Keenan, E.J. Cancer Res. 46: 4237s-4240s, 1986.
28. King, W.J. and Greene, G.L. Nature 307: 745-747, 1984.
29. Welshons, W.V., Lieberman, M.E., and Gorski, J. Nature 307: 747-749, 1984.
30. Martin, P.M. and Sheridan, P.J. J. Steroid Biochem. 16: 215-229, 1982.
31. DeSombre, E.R., Thorpe, S.M., Rose, C., Blough, R.R., Andersen, K.W., Rasmussen, B.B. and King. W.J. Cancer Res. (Suppl) 46: 4256-4264, 1986.
32. Dickson, R.B., McManaway, M.E., and Lippman, M.E. Science 232: 1540-1543, 1986.
33. Toth, J. and DeSombre, E.R. in preparation.
34. Brandes, S.J. and Katzenellenbogen, J.A. Nucl. Med. Biol. 15: 53-67, (1988).
35. Hanson, R.N., Seitz, D.E., and Bottaro, J.C. J. Appl. Radiat. Isot. 35: 810-815, 1984.
36. Pavlik, E.J., Nelson, K., Gallion, H., van Nagell, J.R., Jr., Kenady, D.E., Baranczuk, R.J., Spicer, J. and Preston, D. Abstr. 69th Mtg, Endocrine Soc. p 257, 1987.
37. DeSombre, E.R., Mease, R.C., Sanghavi, J., Singh, T, Seevers, R.H. and Hughes, A. J. Steroid Biochem. 29: 583-590, 1988.
38. Jagoda, E.M., Gibson, R.E., Goodgold, H., Ferreira, N., Francis, B.E., Reba, R.C., Rzeszotarski, W.J., and Eckelman, W.G. J. Nucl. Med. 25: 472-477, 1984.
39. Powell, G.F., DeJesus, O.T., Harper, P.V., and Friedman, A.M. J. Radioanal. Nucl. Chem. Letters 119: 159-170, 1987.
40. Kassis, A.I., Adelstein, S.J., and Bloomer, W.D. In: Radionuclides in Therapy, (eds. R.P. Spencer, R.H. Seevers, and A.M. Friedman) CRC Press, Boca Raton, 1987, pp. 119-134.
41. Bronzert, D.A., Hochberg, R.B., and Lippman, M.E. Endocrinology, 110: 2177-2179, 1982.
42. Nardulli, A.M. and Katzenellenbogen, B.S. Endocrinology 119: 2038-2046, 1986.
43. DeSombre, E.R., Harper, P.V., Hughes, A., Mease, R.C., Gatley, S.J., DeJesus, O.T., and Schwartz, J.L. Cancer Res. 48: 5805-5809, 1988.
44. DeSombre, E.R., Mease, R.C., Hughes, A. Harper, P.V., DeJesus, P.T., and Friedman, A.M. Cancer Res. 48: 899-906, 1988.

14

ESTROGEN INDUCED CATHEPSIN D IN BREAST CANCER : FROM BIOLOGY TO CLINICAL APPLICATIONS

Henri ROCHEFORT, Patrick AUGEREAU, Pierre BRIOZZO, Jean-Paul BROUILLET, Françoise CAPONY, Vincent CAVAILLES, Gilles FREISS, Marcel GARCIA, Thierry MAUDELONDE, Philippe MONTCOURRIER and Françoise VIGNON

Unité Hormones et Cancer (U 148) INSERM and Laboratoire de Biologie Cellulaire, Université de Montpellier, Faculté de Médecine, 60 Rue de Navacelles, 34090 MONTPELLIER France

Susan M. THORPE, Ib J. CHRISTENSEN and Carsten ROSE

University Department of Clinical Physiology and Nuclear Medicine, The Finsen Institute, Rigshospitalet, Strandboulevarden 49, 2100-DK COPENHAGEN Denmark

Estrogens and progestins regulate the growth of hormone responsive breast cancer both _in vitro_ and _in vivo_ (1) and induce several proteins, some of them are likely to play a role in controling the growth, invasiveness and/or differentiation of human breast cancer cells (2-5). We will illustrate how the determination of the structure, functions and regulation of an estrogen-induced secreted protein, the 52K cathepsin D that is isolated from breast cancer cell lines, can lead to clinical applications in breast cancer.

INTRODUCTION

Breast cancer cells are characterized by both their high metastasing capacity and their selective sensitivity to sex steroid hormones. Ten years ago, we decided to use the human breast cancer cell lines MCF7 (6) and T47D (7) which respond to estrogen and progesterone _via_ their own receptors, to define new steroid-induced proteins.

This approach appeared to present several advantages :

1. First, it should facilitate the understanding of the mechanism of action of steroid hormone by allowing the purification of the responsive gene and the study of its regulation in cell culture.

2. By focusing on protein(s) with important biological functions in the growth and spread of breast cancer cells, it could also help in understanding the mechanism by which these hormones regulate the growth and invasiveness of these cancer types.

3. Since the proteins are of human origin, the immunological and genetic probes developped from them will be directly and easily used in clinical studies and could therefore be tested to develop new markers for monitoring breast cancer treatment.

It is now relatively well established that estrogens stimulate the growth of ER+ breast cancer (4-5) while progestin mostly inhibits this growth _via_ its antiestrogenic activity, and also by inducing progestin specific responses. Our laboratory has isolated, identified and cloned a cDNA probe that corresponds to a 250K progestin-induced protein recently identified as the human fatty acid synthetase (18) which may have clinical applications in mammary tissues as described in a separate review (9). In this report, we will concentrate on recent data concerning the biological and clinical significance of the estrogen-induced 52K-cathepsin D.

In 1985, at the same meeting that took place place in London, we reported on a 52K glycoprotein secreted by estrogen-receptor-positive cell lines, induced by estrogens that are able to stimulate the proliferation of the same cells according to an autocrine type mechanism (10). We suggested that this 52K protein might be of interest as a tumor marker and in the process of mammary carcinoge- nesis. During the next 4 years, our laboratory made progress concerning the identification and structure of this protein, the mechanism of its induction, its alteration in cancer cells compared to normal cells, the significance of its proteolytic activity and its relationship with tumor invasion, and finally its usefulness as a prognostic marker in breast cancer patients.

IDENTIFICATION OF THE 52K PROTEIN AS PRO-CATHEPSIN D

The presence of mannose-6-P signals indicated that the protein is normally routed to lysosomes where it exerts its usual function (11). In testing several enzymatic activities that correspond to lysosomal hydrolases of similar molecular weight, we found that both the purified secreted 52K protein and the corresponding cellular proteins (52K, 48K, 34K + 14K) (Fig. 1) displayed a strong proteolytic activity at acidic pH, which was mainly inhibited by pepstatin (12,13). The first 15 amino acids determined by micro-sequencing the N-terminal of the molecules were identical (14).

Fig. 1. Structure of the different molecular forms and processing of cathepsin D. A. Polyacrylamide gel electrophoresis of the purified cathepsin D secreted by MCF7 cells (a) and present in the cell extracts (b). Proteins are revealed after migration by silver staining. In breast cancer cell lines, the proportion of the pro-enzyme (52K) and intermediate (48K) form in the cells is higher than in normal mammary epithelial cells (24).
B. Diagram showing the relationship between these different forms. Secreted pro-cathepsin D can be auto-activated into a 51K form. Intracellularly, pro-cathepsin D is successively maturated in the Golgi, intermediate compartment and lysosomes into an intermediate one-chain-form (48K) and into a two-chain-form (34K + 14K). The intracellular processing requires other proteinases.

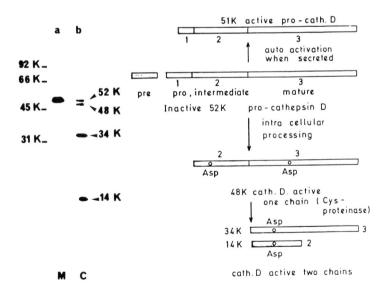

Using both monoclonal antibodies to the secreted 52K protein from MCF7 cells and a synthetic oligonucleotide obtained from partial sequencing of the protein, we screened a λgt11 cDNA library of MCF7 cells kindly given to us by Pierre Chambon (Strasbourg). Four clones (p1-p6-p8 and p9) were isolated and sequenced that covered the whole coding sequence of 52K-mRNA. Comparison of this sequence with that of the pro-cathepsin D of normal human kidneys showed only 5 nucleotide changes giving only one amino acid substitution (Ala to Val) in the pro-fragment (14). It is not yet known whether this change is of general importance in cancer cells or more likely due to a trivial polymorphism since another discrete change was found on cathepsin D cDNA cloned from another RE positive cell line ZR75-1 (15) (Fig. 2).

Fig. 2. Amino acid sequences of human cathepsin D produced by normal tissue and two breast cancer cell lines, deduced from sequencing the corresponding cDNAs: the sequence of pre- pro-cathepsin D from normal human kidney (28), from MCF7 cells (16), and from ZR75-1 cells (17). Four boxes are indicated in the coding region that correspond successively to the signal sequence, the pro-fragment, the short chain of the mature enzyme (14K) and the long chain of the mature enzyme (34K). The positions and type of base modifications are indicated. In MCF7 cells, there is only one amino acid change (Ala to Val) in the pro-fragment (16). In ZR75-1 cells, a different amino acid change (Ala to Thr) in the 34K mature chain was detected in 25% of the cDNA clones (17).

SEQUENCES OF HUMAN CATHEPSIN D

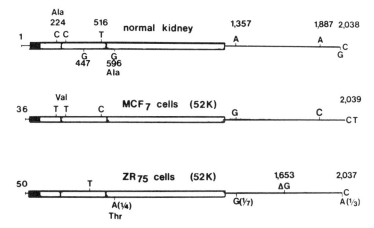

Using in situ hybridization, the gene expressing this protease in normal cells is located on the extremity of the short arm of chromosome 11 close to the H-ras gene (band p15).

TRANSCRIPTIONAL REGULATION OF 52K-CATHEPSIN D BY ESTROGEN AND GROWTH FACTOR

In breast cancer cells, 52K cathepsin D is induced by estrogens, but not by other steroid hormones (16). Estrogens therefore are required for its secretion in RE-positive cancer cells but not in RE-negative cancer cells which produce it constitutively. The 52K- p9 cDNA probe was used to quantify 52K-mRNA by hybridization after Northern blotting. The accumulation of 2.2 kb pre- pro-cathepsin D mRNA was shown to increase approximately 10-fold by estradiol treatment of MCF7 cells but not by tamoxifen (17). This increase is direct and for the most part due to the stimulation of mRNA synthesis at the level of the initiation of transcription as shown by run-on transcription assays. Even though other classes of steroids were inactive, other mitogens such as insulin at high doses, as well as IGF-I, EGF and bFGF can also increase the steady state concentration of cathepsin D-mRNA (18). Thus in breast cancer cells, estrogens can induce both growth factors such as TGF_α and IGF-I (19) and cathepsin D, which can also be induced by these growth factors. The effect of tamoxifen on the 52K cathepsin D gene varies according to the cell line studied (20). In vitro, induction by tamoxifen was seen in the three RE-positive antiestrogen-resistant variants we studied (R27, RTx6 and LY_2). In contrast, tamoxifen acts in vivo within the 3 first weeks of treatment of post-menopausal patients, as an estrogen-agonist for cathepsin D gene expression (21). This increase was probably due to the estrogenic activity of tamoxifen generally observed during the first weeks of treatment that correspond to the flare period. These results indicate that this protease is also induced in vivo by estrogens in breast cancer patients and suggest that this induction may play a role in mediating the effect of estrogens on the proliferative and invasive abilities of breast cancer cells. The stimulation of cathepsin D mRNA expression by several mitogens can be compared to the triggering of cathepsin L mRNA by PDGF and phorbol ester in transformed fibroblasts (22).

ALTERATION OF CATHEPSIN D IN MAMMARY CANCER CELLS

Whereas the normal function of cathepsins takes place in lysosomes at acidic pH, where they degrade endogenous proteins, their increased secretion may have a destructive effect on tissue that surrounds cancer cells. We studied the processing of cathepsin D in normal mammary epithelial cells collected from patients undergoing reduction mammoplasty. These cells were purified after collagenase digestion and cultured on plastic at the same growth rate as MCF7 cells. Pulse chase labeling experiments were performed to quantify cathepsin D-processing (23). As shown in human fibroblasts (24), most of the precursor (52K) was found to be routed to lysosomes and processed rapidly into a mature form (34K + 14K) via the production of an intermediate form (48K) (Fig. 1). Negligible amounts of the pro-form were accumulated in the cells or secreted. In contrast, in several breast cancer cell lines (MCF7, MDA-MB231, BT20, etc), the processing was delayed, the proportion of 52K secretion was markedly increased (up to 50%) and the 52K and 48K forms were accumulated in the cells (23). The increased secretion of pro-cathepsin in cancer cells has also been observed to occur with cathepsin L in transformed fibroblasts (25) and noted with cathepsin B in melanoma (26). A second major difference between normal cells and cancerous ones is that the cytosol concentration of 52K cathepsin D is markedly increased in cancer cells (23). The mechanism of this derouting may be due to a different structure of pro-cathepsin D, which has a lower pI determined by electrofocusing analysis in cancer cells than in normal mammary cells (23). Since the amino acid sequence of the 52K cathepsin D in breast cancer cells is almost identical (except one Ala to Val change) to that of the lysosomal cathepsin D in normal tissues (27), the difference may be due to post-translational modifications and appears to be located on the N-glycosylated chains ; it disappears following removal of the two N-linked oligosaccharides by Endoglycosidase H treatment (23).

PUTATIVE FUNCTIONS IN MAMMARY CARCINOGENENIS

Both biological and clinical studies favor the hypothesis that cathepsin D facilitates critical step(s) in mammary carcinogenesis (28). The derouting of an excess of pro-cathepsin D at the periphery of cancer cells may facilitate cancer cell growth and invasion by digesting basement membrane, extracellular matrix, and connective tissue, and may stimulate cancer cell growth by an autocrine mechanism.

Moreover, a high cathepsin D concentration in intracellular compartments (lysosomes, others ?) may give breast cancer cells a potential advantage in digesting extracellular material and providing a sufficient amount of amino acids to build their own proteins.

In vitro mitogenic activity

In the last 10 years, the concept of estrogen-induced autocrine growth factors secreted by hormone-responsive cancer cells (3) has proved to be very productive. Several estrogen-induced autocrine growth factors have been characterized (19-29) and the purified 52K cathepsin D has been shown to stimulate the growth of estrogen-deprived MCF7 cells (30). Like other proteases, cathepsin D may act indirectly via its enzymatic activity by releasing growth factors from precursors or from cellular matrix and/or by activating growth factor receptors. The alternative is that its mitogenic effect occurs directly via interaction with the mannose-6-phosphate receptor (11) recently identified as the IGF-II receptor (31). Crosslinking and binding experiments have shown that pure 52K pro-cathepsin D interacts directly with the mannose-6-phosphate/IGF-II receptor (M.Mathieu, unpublished experiments). However, the coupling mechanism triggered by the activation of this receptor is unknown and the mechanism and significance of the mitogenic activity of cathepsin D remain mysterious.

In vitro proteolytic activity

Cathepsin D is an aspartyl protease with broad specificity that degrades many proteins (32). The pH required is generally acidic, but can vary according to the substrate. Cathepsin D is secreted as an inactive proenzyme (52K) and can be autoactivated at acidic pH by removing a part of the N-terminal pro-fragment, (14,34) (Fig. 1).

178

Both the purified 52K pro-cathepsin D and conditioned media from estrogen-treated MCF7 cells digest <u>in vitro</u> |³H|proline or |³⁵S| methionine-labeled extracellular matrix prepared from bovine corneal endothelial cells (33). The optimal activity occurs at acidic pH (4 to 5), but not at pH 7. The degradation of extracellular matrix by secreted proteases present in conditioned media is mostly due to cathepsin D, since it was completely inhibited by pepstatin but not by other inhibitors.

<u>Fig. 3.</u> Comparison of the degrading ability of ECM by conditioned media prepared from different cells. Media conditioned by different types of cells, all cultured to subconfluence on plastic, were concentrated 5 times by lyophilization and tested on |³⁵S| methionine-labeled extracellular-matrix at pH 4.5 for 3 days at 37°C. Pepstatin and leupeptin were tested in parallel at 10 μM. Control digestion (medium) was obtained with the respective culture media alone (DEM or RPMI for T47D and BT20 or F12 for normal mammary cells). ECM degradation without (C.M.) and with protease inhibitors (pepst. or leup.) was determined for each cell line according to the release of ³⁵S into the medium. MCF7 R and MCF7 L are the two sublines provided by Drs Marvin Rich and Marc Lippman respectively. (Reprinted with permission from ref. 34).

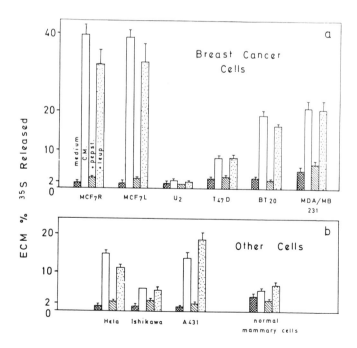

Most cancer cells tested until now secrete a pepstatin-inhibited protease (i.e. aspartyl protease) which appears to be one of the most abundant proteases secreted by epithelial cancer cells (Fig. 3). Moreover, the pepstatin-sensitive protease activities of the different conditioned media correlate perfectly with cathepsin D concentrations in the same C.M., as assayed by ELISA using two specific monoclonal antibodies (33). It is still not known whether secreted pro-cathepsin D can be activated extracellularly under in vivo conditions. This would require an acidic micro-environment which is more frequently encountered in the cells (endosomes, lysosomes, etc...) than out of them. Recently, large acidic vesicles containing both cathepsin D and endocytosed extracellular matrix have been found at a much higher concentration in breast cancer cells compared to normal mammary cells, suggesting that cancer cells display a high phagocytic activity which may be responsible for basement membrane digestion and might explain in part their invasiveness (34).

PROGNOSTIC VALUE OF CATHEPSIN D IN BREAST CANCER PATIENTS

Due to the development of a panel of monoclonal antibodies, total or pro-cathepsin D (52K) can be detected in situ by immuno-peroxidase staining of frozen tissue sections and can be assayed in the cytosol of tumor biopsies using a solid-phase double-determinant immunoassay (ELISA). The results of immunohistochemistry have been reported elsewhere (25,36) ; we will concentrate on the significance of cathepsin D concentration in breast cancer cytosol as measured by ELISA.

Using two combinations of antibodies that recognize two domains of the pro-enzyme (37,38,39), both the pro-cathepsin D (52K) and the total cathepsin D concentration (52K + 48K + 34K) can be assayed in breast cancer cytosol routinely prepared for receptor assays.

The first prospective clinical studies (40,41) have shown that the concentration of cytosolic cathepsin D varies markedly according to the tumor (from 0 to 1,500 pmoles/mg cytosol protein) but is generally higher in breast cancer than in normal mammary glands or benign mastopathies. Using two cut-off levels of about 30 and 60 pmoles/mg cytosol protein, tumors with high, moderate and low cathepsin D level could be defined. Attempts to correlate cathepsin D concentration with classical prognostic parameters have failed for most of them. Cathepsin D concentration was not correlated with estrogen and progesterone receptors or their status. Cathepsin D concentration and status were not correlated with lymph node-invasiveness, tumor size, age of patients, Scarff and Bloom grading (40), or Neu-erb-B-2 and int-2 oncogene amplification (41). A significant correlation was found in pre-menopausal patients between high cathepsin D status and estrogen-receptor-positive tumors in one study (40) and c-myc-oncogene-amplification in another study (41). Hence, from these studies the cytosolic cathepsin D concentration appeared to be an independent parameter. More interesting were the results of a retrospective study allowing the evaluation of the prognostic value of this marker, the clinician being aware of the clinical follow-up of patients during a period of 6 to 7 years. This study was performed in collaboration with the Finsen and Fibiger Institute in Copenhagen (42) and included 150 post-menopausal and 250 pre-menopausal patients of the Danish Breast Cancer Cooperative Group. The cytosol that was collected at surgery six to seven years earlier and kept at -70°C in the Fibiger Center - Finsen Institute was assayed for cathepsin D concentration in Montpellier. In both cases, a significant correlation was found between patients with high cathepsin D concentrations and short recurrence-free survival. The cathepsin D parameter was found to be independent of other prognostic parameters including axillary lymph-node-invasiveness. Fig. 4 illustrates the additive prognostic value of cathepsin D and lymph node invasiveness. Since about 30% of N- patients will relapse, it is crucial to assay at time of surgery other prognostic marker(s) which would help in discriminating these patients (43). Cathepsin D appears to be useful in this respect particularly in N- patients. Fig. 5 shows the prognostic value of cathepsin D status in estrogen receptor and in progesterone receptor positive tumors. In a multiparametric Cox model, the major prognostic factor was lymph-node-invasiveness. The cathepsin D-concentration was the third (post-menopause) or second (pre-menopause) most important parameter, ranking above other classical parameters such as the histopathological grade of the tumour, tumour size, oestrogen receptor, and progesterone receptor (Table 1). Other retrospective studies are in progress independently in the USA and Europe to study the prognostic value of cathepsin D in breast cancer cytosol.

These first clinical studies strongly suggest that cathepsin D plays a role in the process of tumor growth and/or metastasis and should lead to other studies aimed at defining the few best prognostic markers for routine use in breast cancer at the time of surgery, which would allow to define the best therapy.

Fig. 4. Prognostic value of cathepsin D concentration in post-menopausal (a) and pre-menopausal (b) breast cancer patients. In the first retrospective study on 400 patients from the Danish Breast Cancer task force, the total cathepsin D-concentration has been assayed in cytosol, routinely prepared for steroid receptor assays and kept at -70°C for 6-7 years. The assay was blindly made in Montpellier, using a double-determinant ELISA (39) and the relapse-free survival of patients has been registered in Copenhagen in December 1986.

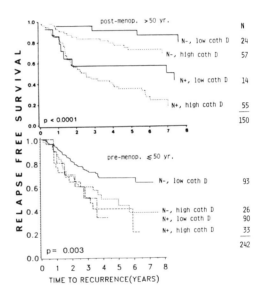

In pre-perimenopausal patients, low cathepsin D concentrations include the first 3 quartiles of the total distribution (i.e. 0-78 pmol/mg cytosol protein).

For the post-menopausal patients, low cathepsin D concentrations include only the first quartile of the total distribution (i.e. 0-24 pmol/mg cytosol protein).

Since the two parameters of node-invasiveness (N-, N+) and cathepsin D status (low, high) are independent, their prognostic value is additive. The number of patients in each group is indicated in the figure.

Table 1.

Final Cox Model - Multivariate Analysis				
	pre/perimenopausal patients (N=242)		post-menopausal patients (N=149)	
Variable	P-value	Relative risk	P-value	Relative risk
Tumor positive lymph nodes (0-3 vs > 4)	0.032	1.79	0.004	2.37
Tumor positive lymph nodes (+ vs -)	-	-	0.012	2.23
Tumor size (+ or - 5 cm)	0.033	1.68	0.004	2.16
Cathepsin-D concentration (low vs high)	0.029	1.68	0.032	1.92
ER status	0.006	0.54	-	-

Criterion for exclusion : $p < 0.10$.
Criterion for secondary inclusion : $p < 0.05$.

Low and high cathepsin D concentrations are defined as described under Fig. 4. The relative risk is based on relapse-free survival as evaluated using the Kaplan-Meier product limit procedure and compared using the log rank test.

CONCLUSIONS AND PERSPECTIVES

It has previously been proposed that proteases are involved in the process of invasion and metastasis by cancer cells (for review, see 44). Collagenases (45) and plasminogen activators have been the most extensively investigated. The tissue type plasminogen activator (46) is also estrogen-regulated in some breast cancer cells; however, its concentration in breast cancer cytosol appears to be associated with a good prognosis (47). The urokinase-type plasminogen activator may be more important in facilitating the tumor invasion process ; however, it is not estrogen-regulated.

Fig. 5. Additional
prognostic value of
cathepsin D concentration
in progesterone or estrogen
receptor positive tumors.
The cathepsin D status is a
prognostic marker independent of estrogen and
progesterone receptors.
These three parameters
therefore appear to be
useful in the assay of the
same cytosol. Primary
breast cancers in 250 pre/
perimenopausal patients
were included. The cut-off
limit for low and high
cathepsin D is 78 pmole/mg
protein in these patients.

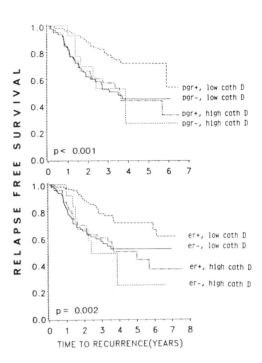

In contrast, cathepsin D is estrogen-induced in RE-positive breast
cancer and produced constitutively in some RE-negative breast
cancers. Its high concentration indicates breast cancer invasiveness
(28,42) and possible high-risk-mastopathy (36). Secreted cathepsin
may therefore be more important than initially anticipated. The
cysteinyl cathepsins (B,L) have been proposed to play a role in some
cancers (25,26) ; pro-cathepsin D appears to be particularly
important in breast cancers and since it is induced by estrogens. It
may also play a role in early steps of mammary carcinogenesis.

Therefore, in hormone-responsive breast cancer, estrogens
increase the coordinated expression of several proteins and peptides
involved in the stimulation of growth and invasiveness, mostly growth
factors and proteases. In estrogen-unresponsive breast cancer, that
corresponds to a later stage of tumor progression, the production of
growth factors and proteases appears to be constitutive. It will be
important to correlate these _in vitro_ studies with more recent
clinical data to specify which step(s) of tumor progression _in vivo_

is (are) favored by an excessive production and secretion of cathepsin D. Contrasting with diagnostic and prognostic applications of cathepsin D in breast cancer, which concern the near future, the therapeutical applications of these studies aimed at inhibiting cathepsin D activity, appear to be more distant. The theoretical advantage of this type of therapy is that it would be efficient in both estrogen receptor positive and negative breast cancer. However, its possible limit is that it might be difficult to inhibit cathepsin D action in cancer cells and not in normal cells. This challenge will require much more time and basic research in the understanding of the molecular mechanism by which the structure, processing and action of cathepsin D differ in normal and cancer cells.

ACKNOWLEDGEMENTS

This work was supported by the "Institut National de la Santé et de la Recherche Médicale", the "Association pour la Recherche sur le Cancer", the School of Medicine and the University Hospital of Montpellier, the "Fédération Nationale des Centres de Lutte contre le Cancer" and the grant INSERM-SANOFI n°81039.3. We thank E. Barrié and M. Egéa for their skillful preparation of the manuscript.

REFERENCES

1. Pike, M.C., Siiteri, P.K. and Welsch, C.W. (eds) Banbury Report 8. Hormones and Breast Cancer, Cold Spring Harbor, Cold Spring Harbor Laboratory, New York, 1981.
2. Sirbasku, D.A. and Benson, R.H. In: Hormones and Cell Culture (Eds. J.H. Sato and R. Ross), Cold Spring Harbor, Cold Spring Harbor Laboratory, Vol. 6, New York, 1979, p. 477.
3. Rochefort, H., Coezy, E., Joly, E., Westley, B. and Vignon, F. In: Hormones and Cancer (Eds. S. Iacobelli, R.J.B. King, H.R. Lindner and M.E. Lippman), Raven Press, Vol. 14, New York, 1980, pp. 21-29.
4. Lippman, M.E., Bolan, G. and Huff, K. Cancer Res. 36:4595-4601, 1986.
5. Chalbos, D., Vignon, F., Keydar, I. and Rochefort, H. J. Clin. Endocrinol. Metab. 55:276-283, 1982.
6. Soule, H.D., Vasquez, J., Lang, A., Albert, S. and Brennan, M.A. J. Natl. Cancer Inst. 51:1409-1413, 1973.
7. Keydar, I., Chen, L., Karby, S., Weiss, F.R., Delarea, J., Radu, M., Chaitcik, S. and Brenner, H.J. Eur. J. Cancer 15:659-670, 1979.
8. Chalbos, D., Chambon, M., Ailhaud, G. and Rochefort, H. J. Biol. Chem. 262:9923-9926, 1987.

9. Chalbos, D., Joyeux, C., Escot, C., Depadova, F. and Rochefort, H. In: Annals of the New York Academy of Sciences, The New York Academy of Sciences, 1989 (in press).
10. H. Rochefort, Capony, F., Cavalié-Barthez, G., Chambon, M., Garcia, M., Massot, O., Morisset, M., Touitou, I., Vignon, F. and Westley, B. In: Breast Cancer : Origins, Detection, and Treatment (Eds. M.A. Rich, J.C. Hager, J. Taylor-Papadimitriou), Martinus Nijhoff Publishing, Boston, 1986, pp. 57-68.
11. Von Figura, K. and Hasilik, A. Ann. Rev. Biochem. 55:167-193, 1986.
12. Capony, F., Morisset, M., Barrett, A.J., Capony, J.P., Broquet, P., Vignon, F., Chambon, M., Louisot, P. and Rochefort, H. J. Cell. Biol. 104:253-262, 1987.
13. Morisset, M., Capony, F. and Rochefort, H. Biochem. Biophys. Res. Commun. 138:102-109, 1986.
14. Augereau, P., Garcia, M., Mattei, M.G., Cavailles, V., Depadova, F., Derocq, D., Capony, F., Ferrara, P. and Rochefort, H. Mol. Endocrinol. 2:186-192, 1988.
15. Westley, B. and May, F.E.B. Nucl. Acids Res. 15:3773-3786, 1987.
16. Westley, B. and Rochefort, H. Cell 20:352-362, 1980.
17. Cavailles, V., Augereau, P., Garcia, M. and Rochefort, H. Nucl. Acids Res. 16:1903-1919, 1988.
18. Cavailles, V., Garcia, M. and Rochefort, H. Mol. Endocrinol. March 1989 (in press).
19. Dickson, R.B., Huff, K.K., Spencer, E.M. and Lippman, M.E. Endocrinology 118:138-142, 1986.
20. Westley, B., May, F.E.B., Brown, A.M.C., Krust, A., Chambon, P., Lippman, M.E. and Rochefort, H. J. Biol. Chem. 259:10030-10035, 1984.
21. Maudelonde, T., Domergue, J., Henquel, C., Freiss, G., Brouillet, J.P., Francès, D., Pujol, H. and Rochefort, H. Cancer 63 April 1989 (in press).
22. Troen, B.R., Gal, S. and Gottesman M.M. Biochem. J. 246:731-735, 1987.
23. Capony, F., Rougeot, C., Montcourrier, P., Cavaillès, V., Salazar, G. and Rochefort, ,H. Submitted for publication.
24. Hasilik, A., Von Figura, K., Conzelmann, E., Nehrkorn, H. and Sandhoff, K. Eur. J. Biochem. 125:317-321, 1982.
25. Gal, S. and Gottesman, M.M. J. Biol. Chem. 261:1760-1765, 1986.
26. Poole, A.R. In: Lysosomes in Biology and Pathology (Eds. J.T. Dingle and H.B. Fell), American Elsevier Pub. Co., New York, 1979, pp. 304-337.
27. Faust, P.L., Kornfeld, S. and Chirgwin, J.M. Proc. Natl. Acad. Sci. USA 82:4910-4914, 1985.
28. Rochefort, H., Capony, F., Garcia, M., Cavailles, V., Freiss, G., Chambon, M., Morisset, M. and Vignon, F. J. Cell. Biochem. 35:17-29, 1987.
29. Lippman, M.E., Dickson, R.B., Bates, S., Knabbe, C., Huff, K., Swain, S., McManaway, M., Bronzert, D., Kasid, A. and Gelmann E.P. Breast Cancer Res. Treat. 1:59-70, 1986.
30. Vignon, F., Capony, F., Chambon, M., Freiss, G., Garcia, M. and Rochefort, H. Endocrinology 118:1537-1545, 1986.
31. Morgan, D.O., Edman, J.C., Standring, D.N., Fried, V.A., Smith, M.C., Roch, R.A. and Rutter, W.J. Nature 329:301-307, 1987.
32. Barett, A.J. Biochem. J. 117:601-607, 1970.

33. Briozzo, P., Morisset, M., Capony, F., Rougeot, C. and Rochefort, H. Cancer Res. 48:3688-3692, 1988.
34. Montcourrier, P., Mangeat, P., Salazar, G., Morisset, M., Sahuquet, A. and Rochefort, H. Submitted for publication.
35. Garcia, M., Salazar-Retana, G., Pages, A., Richer, G., Domergue, J., Pages, A.M., Cavalié, G., Martin, J.M., Lamarque, J.L., Pau, B., Pujol, H. and Rochefort, H. Cancer Res. 46:3734-3738, 1986.
36. Garcia, M., Lacombe, M.J., Duplay, H., Cavailles, V., Derocq, D., Delarue, J.C., Krebs, B., Contesso, G., Sancho-Garnier, H., Richer, G., Domergue, J., Namer, M. and Rochefort, H. J. Steroid Biochem. 27:439-445, 1987.
37. Garcia, M., Capony, F., Derocq, D., Simon, D., Pau, B. and Rochefort, H. Cancer Res. 45:709-716, 1985.
38. Rogier, H., Freiss, G., Besse, M.G., Cavalié-Barthez, G., Garcia, M., Pau, B., Rochefort, H. and Paolucci, F. Clin. Chem. 35:81-85, 1989.
39. Freiss, G., Vignon, F. and Rochefort, H. Cancer Res. 48:3709-3715, 1988.
40. Maudelonde, T., Khalaf, S., Garcia, M., Freiss, G., Duporté, J., Benatia, M., Rogier, H., Paolucci, F., Simony, J., Pujol, H., Pau, B. and Rochefort, H. Cancer Res. 48:462-466, 1988.
41. Brouillet, J.P., Theillet, C., Maudelonde, T., Defrenne, A., Sertour, J. and Rochefort, H. Submitted for publication.
42. Thorpe, S., Rochefort, H., Garcia, M., Freiss, G., Christensen, I.J., Khalaf, S., Paolucci, F., Pau, B., Rasmussen, B.B. and Rose, C. 1989. Submitted for publication.
43. McGuire, W.L. New Engl. J. Med. 320:525-527, 1989.
44. Goldfarb, R.H. In: Mechanisms of Cancer Metastasis (Eds. K.V. Honn, W.E Powers and B.F. Sloane), Martinus Nijhoff Pub., Boston, 1986, pp. 341-375.
45. Liotta, L.A., Tryggvason, K., Garbisa, S., Hart, I., Foltz, C.M. and Shafie, S. Nature 284:67-68, 1980.
46. Butler, W.B., Kirkland, W.L. and Jorgensen, T.L. Biochem. Biophys. Res. Commun. 90:1328-1334, 1979.
47. Duffy, M.J., O'Grady, P. and O'Siorain L. In: Progress in Cancer Research and Therapy, Hormones and Cancer 3 (Eds. F. Bresciani, R.J.B. King, M.E. Lippman and J.P. Raynaud), Raven Press, Vol. 35, New York, 1988, pp. 300-303.

15

CORRELATION BETWEEN THE PRESENCE OF BREAST TUMOR CELLS IN BONE MARROW AT THE TIME OF SURGERY AND DISEASE PROGRESSION

Maria I. Colnaghi
Experimental Oncology E, Istituto Nazionale Tumori, Milano, Italy.

INTRODUCTION

Breast carcinoma is the most alarming form of cancer for women, both in terms of frequency and death rates. In fact, about 40% of patients with an operable tumor develop metastases after surgery, even though the majority of them only show local disease at diagnosis according to staging by conventional methods. This seems to suggest that, on presentation, a certain number of patients already have disseminated disease, which however cannot be revealed by our current methods of detection. Reliable factors capable of predicting which patients will develop metastatic cancer and when, are not yet available. Prognosis seems to be correlated, to a certain extent, with some parameters identified by clinical, pathological and biochemical studies, such as clinical stage, nodal status and hormone receptor levels. However, none of them are entirely dependable. Today there is still an urgent need to discover new tools which can help us identify those subgroups of patients which undergo a different course of disease and subsequently require different treatment.

The skeleton is a common site for metastases in breast cancer and at present, possible bone marrow involvement is being investigated by radiologic, scintigraphic or hematologic techniques, none of which are sensitive enough to reveal very slight bone marrow contamination, particularly if the involvement is limited to isolated tumor cells. The combined use of immunologic and histochemical methods and the exploitation of monospecific reagents, such as monoclonal antibodies (MAbs), for discriminating tumor cells from normal ones of a different histogenetical origin, has greatly improved detection sensitivity so that even a single tumor cell can easily be identified on a slide preparation.

This paper reviews the results of 4 studies aimed at evaluating the usefulness of immunohistochemistry for revealing possible occult micrometastases in bone marrow biopsies harvested at the time of surgery from operable breast cancer patients and determining the prognostic value of this approach.

RESULTS

Following the study at the Ludwig Institute and Royal Marsden in London (1), three other trials have been carried out (2-4). The reagents used for the immunologic tests were: an antiserum to epithelial membrane antigen being raised in rabbits against human milk fat globule membrane (1); an anti-cytokeratin-component-18 MAb (2); a pool of 3 mouse MAbs reacting with distinct epithelial antigens (3); a mouse MAb reacting with normal and transformed epithelial mammary cells (4). No reactivity was observed, for each of the MAbs used, with normal or neoplastic bone marrow cells. In the case of the antiserum, a weak non-specific staining of normal bone marrow cells, in particular plasma cells, was noted (5,6). In this case, therefore, the immunostained cells were considered positive provided that they conformed to the identification of tumor cells on morphological grounds (7).

The sensitivity of the immunologic test was found to be superior to that of conventional methods. Among the total 365 bone marrow samples from breast cancer patients evaluated in the Munich, New York and Milan studies using MAbs, i.e. reagents absolutely reliable in terms of specificity, immunoreactive cells were identified in 71 samples, whereas none of the 365 cases were found to be contaminated by tumor cells according to conventional cytology or histology (Table 1).

Table 1.

EPITHELIAL TUMOR CELLS IN BONE MARROW: CONVENTIONAL HISTOLOGY AND CYTOLOGY COMPARED WITH IMMUNOCYTOLOGY

Authors	No. positive cases/Total no. cases (%)	
	Conventional techniques	Immunocytology
Schlimok (87)	0/155 (0)	28/155 (18)
Cote (88)	0/ 51 (0)	18/ 51 (38)
Porro (88)	0/159 (0)	25/159 (16)
Total	0/365 (0)	71/365 (19)

The fine degree of sensitivity was evaluated in the Milan study by analyzing the ability of the MAb MBr1 to detect a known amount of breast carcinoma cells artificially mixed with an excess of human leukocytes. The test was demonstrated to be sensitive enough to reveal tumor cells at a concentration level as low as one out of 200,000 leukocytes (4). In this study, to facilitate the differentiation of normal cells from tumor ones, the latter were stained with bisbenzimide before being added at different concentrations, from 5 to 320, to 1×10^6 living leukocytes. The cell suspensions were then examined by indirect immunofluorescence after MBr1 MAb labelling. None of the unstained bisbenzimide cells were stained by fluorescein, thus confirming the non-reactivity of MBr1 MAb with cells of hemapoietic origin.

Analogous results were obtained by Schlimok et al. who, to exclude a spurious reaction of the anti-cytokeratin MAb with hemopoietic cells, used a double staining procedure that included an anti-leukocyte-common-antigen MAb. In all of the tested samples no cells were found to be positive with both MAbs (2).

Table 2

DETECTION OF OCCULT METASTASES IN BONE MARROW ASPIRATES OF
BREAST CANCER PATIENTS

No. cases	No. cases with immunopos. cells	Reagent	Author
307	81 (26%)	As α EMA	Mansi et al., 1987
155	28 (18%)	MAb CK2	Schlimok et al., 1987
51	18 (35%)	MAb pool	Cote et al., 1988
159	25 (16%)	MAb MBr1	Porro et al., 1988
Total 672	152 (23%)		

Table 2 summarizes the data regarding the detection of occult tumor cells in bone marrow aspirates, obtained by the 4 groups. Immunoreactive cells were found in percentages varying from 16 to 35% out of the total number of 672 breast cancer patients evaluated. These different percentages could be attributed to the different sensitivity of the reagents used and to the different stages of the disease of the patients which entered the various trials. For example, in the Milan study all the patients were clinically N0 or N1a, whereas in the New York trial patients in advanced stages were also included. Moreover, in our study we used a MAb which is able to recognize only 80% of breast carcinoma, a detection efficiency which is lower than that of the anti-cytokeratin MAb or the pool of MAbs.

The London group reported results concerning the analysis of bone marrow samples from 307 patients with primary breast carcinoma (1). Micrometastases were found in 26% of the cases studied and their presence was related to various poor prognostic factors, such as lymph node involvement, pathological size and vascular invasion. After a median follow-up of 28 months, 60 patients relapsed at distant sites. The analysis of the sites of relapse showed that the test predicted bone metastases only. Among patients who developed bone metastases, 53% had immunologically detected micrometastases at presentation, compared with only 14% of those who remained disease-free or relapsed in non-skeletal sites.

The Munich study (2) includes 155 patients with breast cancer. Tumor cells were detected in 9% of patients without distant metastases and in 19% of the total number of patients examined. A significant correlation was found between the presence of tumor cells in the bone marrow and conventional risk factors. Preliminary results of the follow-up (personal communication), indicate a strong correlation between bone marrow immunoreactivity and poor prognosis. In fact, 82% of the bone marrow positive patients relapsed versus 11% of the bone marrow negative patients (median follow-up: 31 months).

In the New York study (3), extrinsic cells were found in the bone marrow of 35% of the 51 patients with operable breast carcinoma. The presence of these micrometastases did not correlate with tumor size or lymphatic invasion around the tumor. The lymph node status showed a trend to correlate with the presence of epithelial antigen positive cells in the bone marrow. However, no statistical significance could be attributed to this trend, considering the limited amount of case material which was evaluated. The same view also concerns the follow-up: the number of patients (41) is too small for any statistically significant results to be obtained. However, a shorter relapse time and a greater percentage of relapses were observed in bone marrow positive patients (personal communication).

In our study, cell suspensions of 159 bone marrow biopsies, harvested at the time of surgery from T1T2N0M0 breast cancer patients, were analyzed and 25 of them were found to contain MBr1 reactive cells. Among the 101 cases confirmed N- pathologically, 17 samples showed MBr1-reactive cells. Conventional histological examination of the same bone marrow samples did not reveal any tumor cells. The similar distribution of bone marrow contaminating tumor cells which was found in N+ and N- patients is due to the fact that in our study N+ patients were actually clinically lymph node negative, i.e. the lymph node contamination was very limited. It is known that a sharp rise in the relapse rate only occurred when 4 or more axillary nodes were involved (8). Preliminary results of the follow-up, evaluated in 121 cases, (median 45 months), reported in Table 3, indicate that the percentage of relapse in patients with immunologically positive bone marrow was significantly higher than that of bone marrow negative patients (40% versus 20%). As opposed to results obtained by the London group, the predictivity in our case was not limited to skeletal recurrence.

Table 3

CORRELATION BETWEEN THE PRESENCE OF MBr1-POSITIVE CELLS IN THE BONE MARROW THE AT TIME OF SURGERY AND THE DEVELOPMENT OF METASTASES

MBr1-positive cells in the bone marrow	Total no. of cases	No. of relapsed patients	%
yes	20	8	40*
no	101	20	20*

p = 0.05

In Table 4 the results of the 4 studies are considered together in order to evaluate in a large number of patients the prognostic significance of the immunoreactive cells in the bone marrow. Among the 558 evaluated patients, tumor cells were identified in 41% of the relapsed patients versus 18% of patients with no evidence of disease, a difference which is statistically significant (logistic regression model: odds ratio = 3.13).

Beyond the results of the single trials, some of which possibly include too few patients for results to be considered statistically significant, the overall analysis of the various studies which altogether take into account an adequate number of cases, indicates that this approach may prove to be a useful and sensitive tool to monitor patients in order to identify an at risk population that at present cannot be revealed by current methods of detection.

Table 4

CORRELATION BETWEEN THE PRESENCE OF IMMUNOREACTIVE CELLS IN THE BONE MARROW AT THE TIME OF SURGERY AND RELAPSE. SUMMARY OF THE STUDIES AT THE 4 CENTERS

| Center | No. of cases | Follow-up | | | |
| | | NED | | ED | |
		b.m.+(%)	b.m.-(%)	b.m.+(%)	b.m.-(%)
London	307	55 (22)	192 (78)	26 (43)	34 (57)
Munich	89	2 (3)	69 (97)	9 (50)	9 (50)
New York	41	10 (32)	21 (68)	4 (40)	6 (60)
Milan	121	12 (13)	81 (87)	8 (29)	20 (71)
Total	558	79 (18)	363 (82)	47 (41)	69 (59)

Logistic regression model: odds ratio: 3.13 (2.01 - 4.87)

In our case, the criteria for selecting, for this approach, a reagent which is unable to identify the totality of breast carcinoma histotypes, was based on the results of a retrospective study which indicated that the expression on tumor cells of the molecule recognized by the MBr1 MAb is associated with a poor prognosis (9). In this particular study, and in a more recent one (unpublished results), MBr1, due to its persistent reactivity on paraffin-embedded sections, was tested on histological tumor samples in order to evaluate a possible relationship between the presence of the relevant antigens on the primary tumors and disease progression. The heterogeneous expression of the antigen identified by the reagent on the carcinomas made this MAb a suitable candidate for analysis regarding its predicting potential. The study was carried out using the immunoperoxidase test on histologic sections from surgical specimens. The overall case material included tumor samples from 100 breast carcinoma patients, in all stages of the disease, all of which, in follow-up for at least 5 years, relapsed. The survival after 5 years was 29% for the group of patients whose primary tumors were MBr1-positive and 63% for the patients whose tumors were MBr1-negative.

On the basis of these results it was possible to hypothesize that the presence in the bone marrow of MBr1-positive cells could have a predicting potential superior to that associated with the presence of tumor cells identified by reagents which simply recognize an epithelial origin.

The final results of the follow-up at the various centers should clarify this point.

REFERENCES

1. Mansi, J.L., Berger, U., Easton, D., McDonnell, T., Redding, W.H., Gazet, J.C., McKinna, A., Powles, T.J., Coombes, R.C. Br. Med. J. 295: 1093-1096, 1987.

2. Schlimok, G., Funke, I., Holzmann, B., Göttlinger, G., Schmidt, G., Häuser, H., Swierkot, S., Warnecke, H.H., Schneider, B., Koprowski, H., Riethmüller, G. Proc. Natl. Acad. Sci. 84: 8672-8676, 1987.

3. Cote, R.J., Rosen, P.P., Hakes, T.B., Sedira, M., Bazinet, M., Kinne, D.W., Old, L.J., Osborne, M.P. Am. J. of Surg. Pathol. 12: 333-340, 1988.

4. Porro, G., Ménard, S., Tagliabue, E., Orefice,S., Salvadori, B., Squicciarini, P., Andreola, S., Rilke, F., Colnaghi, M.I. Cancer 61: 2407-2411, 1988.

5. Delsol, G., Gatter, K.C., Stein, H., Erber, W.N., Pulford, K.A.F., Zinne, K., Mason, D.Y. Lancet ii 1124-1128, 1984.

6. Sloane, J.P., Dearnaley, D.P., Ormerod, M.G. Lancet ii 109-110, 1985.

7. Dearnaley, D.P., Sloane, J.P., Ormerod, M.G., Steele, K., Coombes, R.C., Clink, H.McD., Powles, T.J., Ford, H.T., Gazet, J.C., Neville, A.M. Br. J. Cancer 44: 85-90, 1981.

8. Saez, R.A., Clark, G.M., McGuire, W.L. In: Baillière's Clinical Oncology. Breast Cancer. (Ed. U. Veronesi) vol. 2 pp 103-115, 1988.

9. Colnaghi, M.I. In: Baillière's Clinical Oncology. Breast Cancer. (Ed. U. Veronesi) vol. 2 pp 85-102, 1988.

16

THE GROWING IMPORTANCE OF PRE-INVASIVE CARCINOMA OF
THE BREAST

PAULINE G. HECHT, M.D., F.A.C.S.

Director of Surgical Oncology, New York Infirmary-
Beekman Downtown Hospital, New York City, U.S.A.

Pre-invasive breast cancer has been described
and recognized as an entity for many years. Until
recently, it has been considered relatively unimpor-
tant. These pre-invasive lesions, also known as carcinoma in situ, were formerly reported as comprising
only 1-2% of all breast cancer[1,2]. However, analysis
of recent statistics discloses the growing importance
of these lesions. Mainly as the result of the prevalence of mammographic screening, these in situ carcinomas are found to make up over 20% of mammographic-
ally diagnosed minimal breast cancers[3]. Refinements
in mammographic technology permit not only an earlier
diagnosis of all cancers of the breast, but in particular, of the in situ forms. Now that we see more of
these pre-invasive cancers (Fig. 1), we can analyze
them histologically and study their behavior. Mammographic diagnosis reveals the presence of the suspect
microcalcifications (Fig. 2), and operative radiographic monitoring assures the complete excision of the
lesions in question (Fig. 3).

PERSONAL SERIES - BREAST SURGERY
1988

Benign Lesions   189
Infiltrating Carcinoma 39
Lobular Carcinoma in
        situ   6
Ductal Carcinoma in
        situ   5

Fig. 1. Personal series, one year, reflecting
relative high proportion of in situ
carcinomas.

Carcinoma in situ of the mammary lobules arises
in the cells of the acini and terminal ducts. Most of
the acini within a lobule are involved. The lobules
may be of normal size or enlarged, with irregular hyperplasia of the lining cells, until the lumen is
plugged (Figs. 4 and 5) The lesion is frequently
microscopically discovered as a coincidental companion
to other breast pathology for which biopsy is being

performed.

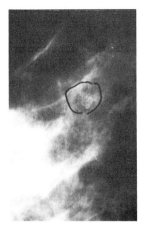

Fig. 2.
Typical Microcalcifica-
tions on Mammography.

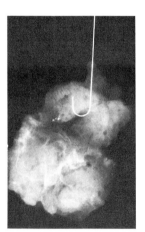

Fig. 3.
Excision of Microcalcifi-
cations Radiographically
Confirmed on Xray of
Operative Excsion Specimen.

The two significant features of lobular carcinoma
in situ are its multifocal appearance in the involved
breast, and its tendency to be bilateral. Studies
of breast specimens removed for lobular carcinoma in
situ showed that 88% of the breasts had other foci of
lobular carcinoma in situ scattered throughout the
specimen (4). Examination of contralateral breast
biopsies has shown in situ lobular carcinoma in from
35 to 59 % (5).

Haagenson, who does not accept lobular carcinoma
in situ as a malignant lesion, and prefers to call it
lobular neoplasia, has clearly demonstrated that lobular carcinoma in situ is a marker which identifies

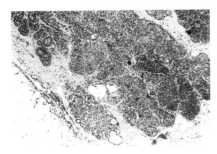

Fig. 4.
Lobular Carcinoma in Situ,
Low Power.

Fig. 5.
Lobular Carcinoma in
Situ, higher magnifica-
tion, showing filling of
lobular lumina with cell-
ular proliferation.

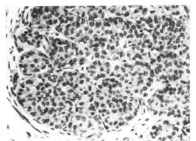

the high risk patient, who will develop breast cancer,
(6). Other investigators have confirmed that this
specific pre-invasive lesion carries the risk of development of invasive cancer with equal frequency in
either breast, in patients followed 25 years or
longer (7).

The other form of pre-invasive breast carcinoma
is ductal carcinoma in situ, also known as intraductal
carcinoma.

In ductal carcinoma in situ, the duct epithelium
is usually thrown up into papillae which show dis-
orientation of cells, with pleomorphism, and occasionally mitotic figures, but without evidence of invasion
of the basement membrane (Gigs. 6 and 7).

Ductal carcinomas in situ are subdivided into
four groups: Comedo, Cribriform- with or without necrosis, Cribriform with anaplasia, and Papillary
Fig . 8). This classification is based on analysis of
cyto-architecture and presence or absence of necrosis (8).

Recent study of these sub-groups of ductal carcinoma in situ reveals correlation between their
growth and invasiveness and their cell type and size
of lesion (Figs. 9 and 10). Recurrences are more
frequently seen in comedo and cribriform than in

micropapillary variants (8), and in lesions over 25 mm. in diameter (8). Further classification and correlation with clinical behavior is based on analysis of nuclear grade and DNA cytometry.

Fig. 6.
Ductal Carcinoma in Situ,
Low Magnification.

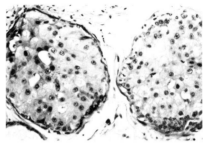

Fig. 7.
Ductal Carcinoma in Situ,
Higher Magnification,
Showing Intact Basement
Membrane.

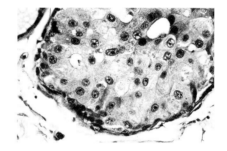

In contrast to lobular carcinoma in situ, ductal carcinoma in situ is associated with recurrences and with the appearance of invasive ductal carcinoma in the same breast. These develop either from incomplete resection of previously recognized involvement, or from an unsuspected focus in the same breast.

Total mastectomy is virtually curative for ductal in situ carcinoma. But current focus on breast conservation creates a dilemma. Whether procedures less than mastectomy will suffice for intraductal carcinoma is of great concern. This concern is triggered by the finding of axillary nodal metastatic involvement in 2% of patients treated by modified radical mastectomy, implying the synchronous presence of an undiagnosed or unrecognized invasive component in the breast with the ductal carcinoma in situ (9).

We hope that by analyzing the nuclear grade, cyto-architecture, presence or absence of necrosis,

DNA cytometry, and with post-operative mammographic control to ensure excision of all lesions, we will be able to select that group of patients with ductal carcinoma in situ who could be treated safely with simple excision and breast conservation.

In summary, the growing absolute number and proportion of pre-invasive cancers demands an increased awareness on our part of the significance of these lesions. We must learn their specific patterns of behavior, so that we may precisely individualize our therapy for patients with pre-invasive breast cancer.

BIBLIOGRAPHY

1. Schwartz, S.I., Shires,G.T., Spencer, F., Storer,E.H Principles of Surgery, 1979.

2. Rosen, P.P. The Pathological Classification of Human Mammary Carcinoma: Past, Present, and Future. Ann. Clin. Lab. Sci., 1979, 9: 144-156.

3. Baker, L.H. Breast Cancer Demonstration Project: Five Year Summary Report, CA 1982, 32: 194-225.

4. Hutter, R.V.P., Foote, F.W., Farrow, J.H. In Situ Lobular Carcinoma of the Female Breast, 1939-1968. Proceedings of the 13th Annual Clinical Conference, Breast Cancer Early and Late. University of Texas, M.D. Anderson Hospital and Tumor Institute of Houston. Yearbook Medical Publishers, Chicago, 1970: 201-226.

5. Rosen, P.P., Lieberman, P.H., Braun, D.W.,Kosloff,C. Adair, F. Lobular Carcinoma in Situ of the Breast: Detailed Analysis of 99 Patients with Average Follow-up of 24 Years. Am. J. Surg. Path., 1978, 2: 225-251.

6. Haagensen, C.D., Bodian, C., Haagensen, D. Breast Carcinoma- Risk and Detection. W. B. Saunders, 1981, 289.

7. Ibid., 1981, 267.

8. Lagios, M.D., Margolin, F.R, Westdahl, P.H.,Rose,M.R Cancer, 1989, 63: 618-624.

9. Rosen, P.P., Braun, D.W., Kinne, D.E. Cancer, 46: 919-925, 1980.

17

ROLE OF DIET IN BREAST CANCER ETIOLOGY

BARUCH MODAN, M.D., and FLORA LUBIN, B.Sc.

Department of Clinical Epidemiology, Chaim Sheba Medical Center, Tel Aviv University Medical School, Tel Hashomer, Israel.

Like many other ideas that are considered innovative, the beneficial effect of vegetarian diet goes back to the Bible. More than 2500 years ago Daniel (1) convinced his Persian captors, who had almost forced him and his three friends to keep high fat carnivorous diet, that their subsistence on grains was preferential. Indeed, ten days later they looked better and healthier than the native children. Needless to say, the sample size was small, the follow up period short, the findings could have resulted from a multitude of confounders, and the study did not receive the approval of an Institutional Review Board. Still, this biblical episode can be envisaged as a first anecdotal piece of information for the advantage of fiber over fat.

That diet may be involved in cancer etiology was first directly reported at the turn of the century by Rollo Russell (2), who stated that in "countries that eat more flesh" cancer mortality is higher. Experimental investigations became abundant already in the 1940's, and the subject received special impetus over the past quarter of a decade. Yet, it was only in the mid Nineteen Seventies

that the US National Cancer Institute started to involve

the scientific community in the search for a dietary role

in breast cancer etiology.

Figure 1

Sources for Current State of Information
on Nutrition in Breast Cancer Causality

Experimental (animals)
  Fat   Occasional Carcinogens
  Fiber
  Energy

 Correlation of   Changes in Incidence
Mortality Incidence   Time
with Dietary Patterns   Migration

Analytical Dietary Studies:
  1) Case-control
  2) Cohort

Positive Associations   Negative Association
  Fat   Vitamin C,A & Fiber
  Alcohol?

Experimental (human)
  Intervention
  ???

Current evidence for the relationship of diet to the

etiology of breast cancer (Fig. 1) is based on three types

of data: a) laboratory experimentation, b) indirect relation-

ships between consumption of selected nutrients and cancer

incidence or mortality in specific geographic regions, and

c) analytical studies in humans.

Experimental evidence

The experimental evidence has focused primarily on three areas: identification of carcinogenic agents, (3-12), definition of metabolic pathways promoting or modifying the behavior of known carcinogens (13-18), and description of a potentially protective mechanism (19). The studies have indicated primarily a promoting effect of fat and higher energy intake, and to a lesser extent on an inhibitory effect of restricted caloric diet, fiber, and vitamins A, C, and E.

Any attempt to extrapolate carcinogenic mechanisms from animals to humans must take into account the problems of dosage, the fact that laboratory experimentation can be based on individual nutrients, and the differing threshold needed for a proven carcinogen to be effective in man. Experimental data in humans are limited to a small number of intervention studies, primarily of high risk groups with emphasis on low fat diet. These, however, have not been completed.

Indirect Relationships

Observed relationships between the consumption of selected nutritional constituents and breast cancer incidence and mortality include the following:
1. Quantified positive correlations between per capita fat consumption and breast cancer mortality or morbidity (20-24), and an inverse correlation with complex carbohydrates (25).

2. Associations between nutritional patterns based on individual dietary histories of women in high or low risk populations, meatless diet of Seventh Day Adventists, or the hormonal profile of vegetarian women (26-32).

3. Time trends in breast cancer incidence that parallel differences in consumption trends (33); i.e. increasing incidence in afluent societies.

4. Observed changes in disease incidence among migrants. For instance, gradually increasing rates in Japanese-Americans (34).

Analytical Studies

Results of 11 such studies are summarized in Table 1 (35-46). The data are inconsistent: about four of the reported studies indicate excess of fat consumption, while seven do not. By the same token, only a minority of the studies report a protective effect of fiber or vitamins. Lately, alcohol has been found to be positively associated with breast cancer. However, this association is incon-clusive since the number of studies implicating alcohol approximates those that do not (47-53).

Our own data (41) indicate that fat, animal protein and fiber do play a combined role in post menopausal breast cancer etiology. This conclusion is based on a case-control study on 818 breast cancer patients and two matched controls groups, surgical and neighborhood, diag-nosed in Israel between 1976 and 1978. The interview schedule included a full dietary history, based on the

Table 1. Summary of findings from selected nutritional analytical studies of breast cancer

Author and Reference	Population and Location	Study Population	Fat	Fiber, Fruits, Vegetables	Vit.A/ Caroten
Philips (35)	CA, Seventh Day Adventists (1975)	77 cases 77 controls(P)	+	N.A.	N.A.
Miller et al. (36)	Canada (1977)	400 cases 400 controls(P)	+	N.A.	N.A.
Graham et al. (37)	Buffalo (1982)	2024 cases 1463 controls(S)	N.D.	N.D.	-
J. Lubin & Burns (38)	Alberta (1982)	577 cases 826 controls(P)	+	N.A.	N.A.
Philips & Snowden (39)	CA, Seventh Day Adventist (1983)	21,295 186 cases	N.D.	N.A.	N.A.
Katsouyanni et al. (46)	Greece (1986)	120 cases 120 controls(S)	N.D.	-	-
F. Lubin et al (41)	Israel (1987)	818 cases 743 controls(S) 813 controls(P)	+	-	N.A.
Jones et al. (42)	USA (NHANES) (1987)	5,485 99 cases	N.D.	N.D.	N.A.
Willet et al. (43)	MA (Nurses) (1987)	89,538 601 cases	N.D.	N.D.	N.D.
Hirohata et al. (44)	Hawaii (1987)	183 cases (J) 183 controls(S) 183 controls(P)	N.D.	N.A.	N.A.
		161 cases (C) 161 controls(S) 161 controls(P)	N.D.	N.A.	N.A.
Rohan & Bain (45)	Australia (1988)	451 cases 451 controls(P)	N.D.	N.D.	-
Marubini et al. (46)	Milan (1988)	214 cases 215 controls(S)	N.A.	N.A.	-

+ = positive association   (P) = population
- = negative association   (S) = surgical
NA = not ascertained;   (J) = Japanese
ND = not determined   (C) = Caucasian

frequency of consumption of 250 food items, grouped according to their principal nutrient component.

There was a trend of increased risk with increased fat
and animal protein, and a decreased fiber intake, at a
p value of .10 and .02 for pre- and post-menopausal women
respectively (Table 2). Similar results were obtained when
fruit and vegetable subgroups were substituted for all
foods containing fiber. Yet, these findings are not as
strong as the clear demonstration of the protective role
of fiber observed by us previously for colon cancer, when
a similar methodology was used.

Table 2. Adjusted relative risk (RR) of breast cancer for
patterns of combined consumption of fat, animal protein
and fiber, by approximate menopausal state (41)

			AGE GROUP	
			≤50	50+
LEVELS OF CONSUMPTION				
Fat	Animal Protein	Fiber	RR*	RR*
Lowest	Lowest	High	1.00	1.00
Low	Low	Intermediate	.83	1.33
Intermediate	Intermediate	Low	1.43	1.38
High	High	Lowest	1.59 (.5,4.6)	1.99 (1.1,3.7)
One-tailed p value for linear trend			.10	.02

* 95% confidence intervals are given in parentheses

DISCUSSION

Dietary studies have been criticized for an inaccuracy due to deficient recall, inaccuracy in quantification, and an inability to determine the relative diet at the time of onset of the carcinogenic process.

The most crucial criteria for the acceptance of dietary information as etiologic are consistency of results. This, however, has become a rare event.

The reasons for the inconsistency between the various analytic studies of breast cancer could stem from the following factors:

1) Limited and/or uneven list of food items

2) Differences in type of controls selected

3) Uncertainty with regard to the relationship between the time period surveyed and the patients' actual age at tumor induction

4) Lack of distinction between pre- and post menopausal phases of breast cancer in some of the studies

5) Methodological flaws

6) The fact that positive findings are more publishable than negative ones

7) A limited effect

Long term prospective studies do not provide an optimal alternative. If, indeed, recent diet is not representative of the individual's long term nutritional patterns, then obtaining dietary information at one particular point of time may not be indicative and does not ensure against future changes. The conflicting findings between the one prospective study (43) and those where a retrospective approach was used, should not be construed as a proof for the invalidity of retrospectively obtained data. In the particular prospective study, which is now considered by some as a major argument against the presence of a fat or fiber effect in breast carcinogenesis, most of the subjects were pre-menopausal at the presumptive outcome; also the time interval between initial interview and cancer diagnosis was relatively short.

It seems, that if there is a true dietary role in breast carcinogenesis it is of a borderline magnitude at most. If so, why has the role of diet achieved such a prominent place in preventive oncology?

There are at least three factors that provide an explanation to this provocative question.

1. Breast cancer incidence is strongly related to socio-economic status and therefore it is on the rise in all developed countries. The current pattern of marrying late and delaying first delivery, will doubtless contribute to even higher incidence in the future. Therefore, it has become a disease that presents a major threat to our society.

2. There is very little one can do to combat breast cancer. Of the four main risk factors - genetic suscepti-bility, radiation, hormonal profile, and diet - only the latter one is amenable to some kind of modification.

Radiation exposure is already being decreased as much as possible, and the balance is hardly controllable (background, Chernobyl, therapeutic). By the same token, one can do practically nothing against genetic traits and very little to delay menarche, or to persuade the younger generation to bear children at an earlier age. Thus, diet remains the only hopeful outreach program in the quest for prevention.

3. Even a small diminishing effect on a highly prevalent disease can yield a considerable absolute yield.

CONCLUSION

Current evidence for the involvement of diet in cancer etiology is based on laboratory data, correlations between the consumption of selected food constituents and incidence, as well as analytic dietary studies. The most likely dietary causative pattern, if any, is the combination of high-fat - low-fiber consumption, that bears an inter-relationship with hormonal metabolism. It seems however that the high hopes of dietary control of breast cancer have been only partly accomplished.

On the other hand, a prudent low-fat high-fiber diet is beneficial in reducing the incidence of a whole spectrum of modern diseases. The idea of a potentially partial dietary control of breast cancer should therefore not be totally abandoned prematurely.

REFERENCES

1. Daniel 1,12-16.
2. Russell, R. Note on the causation of cancer. Longmans, London, 1916, 116 pp.
3. Visscher, M.B., Ball, Z.B., Barnes, R.H., et al. Surgery 11:48-55, 1942.
4. Tannenbaum, A. Cancer Res. 2:468-475, 1942.
5. Carroll, K.K., and Hopkins, G.J. Lipids 14:155-158, 1979.
6. Welsch, C.W., and Aylsworth, C.F. JNCI. 70:215-221, 1983.
7. Rao, G.A., and Abraham, S. JNCI 56:431-432, 1976.
8. Carroll, K.K., and Khor, H.T. Cancer Res. 30:2260-2264, 1970.
9. Kritchevsky, D., Weber, M.M., and Klurfeld, D.M. Cancer Res. 44:3174-3177, 1984.
10. Boissonneault, G.A., Elson, C.E., and Pariza, M.W. JNCI. 76:335-338, 1986.
11. Dunning, W.F., Curtis, M.R., and Maun, M.E. Cancer Res. 9:354-361, 1949.
12. Tannenbaum, A. Cancer Res. 5:609-615, 1945.
13. Hill, M.J., Goddard, P., and Williams, R.E.O. Lancet 2:472-473, 1971.
14. Chan, P.C., and Cohen, L.A. J. Natl. Cancer Inst. 52:25- 30, 1974.
15. Ip, C., Yip, P.H. and Bernadis, L.L. Cancer Res. 40:374-378, 1980.
16. Goldin, B.R., Adlergreutz, H., Dwyer, J.T, et al. Cancer Res. 41:3771-3773, 1981.
17. Anderson, K.E., Kappas, A., Conney, A.H., Bradlow, H.L., and Fishman, J. J. Clin. Endocrinol. Metab. 59:103-107, 1984.
18. Papatestas, A.E., Panvelliwalla, D., Tartter, P.I., et al. Cancer 49:1201-1205, 1982.
19. Adlercreutz, H. Gastroenterology 86:761-766, 1984.
20. Drasar, B.S., and Irving, D. Br. J. Cancer 27:167-172, 1973.
21. Armstrong, B., and Doll, R. Int. J. Cancer 15:617-631, 1975.
22. Correa, P. Cancer Res. 41:3685-3690, 1981.
23. Gray, G.E., Pilse, M.C., Henderson, B.E. Br. J. Cancer 39:1-7, 1979.
24. Gaskill, S.P., McGuire, W.L., Osborne, C.K., et al. Cancer Res. 39:3628-3637, 1979.
25. Hems, G., and Stuart, A. Br. J. Cancer 31:118-123, 1975.
26. Armstrong, B.K., Brown, J.B., Clarke, H.T., et al. JNCI. 67:761-767, 1981.
27. Goldin, B.R., Adlercreutz, H., Gorbach, S.L., et al. N. Engl. J. Med. 307:1542-1547, 1982.
28. Shultz, T.D., and Leklem, J.E. Nutr. Cancer 4:247-259, 1983.

29. Kolonel, L.N., Hankin, J.H., Nomura, A.M., et al. Cancer Res. 41:3727-3728, 1981.
30. Talamini, R., La Vecchia, C., Decarli, A., et al. Br. J. Cancer 49:723-239, 1984.
31. Dunn, J.E., Jr. Cancer Res. 35:3240-3245, 1975.
32. Goldin, B.R., Adlercreutz, H., Gorbach, S.L., et al. Am. J. Clin. Nutr. 44:945-953, 1986.
33. Hirayama, T. Prev. Med. 7:173-195, 1978.
34. Buell, P. J. Natl. Cancer Inst. 51:1479-1483, 1973.
35. Philips, R.L. Cancer Res. 35:3513-3522, 1975.
36. Miller, A.B., Kelly, A., Choi, N.W., et al. Am. J. Epidemiol. 107:499-509, 1978.
37. Graham, S., Marshall, J., Mettlin, C., et al. Am. J. Epidemiol. 116:68-75, 1982.
38. Lubin, J.H., Burns, P.E., Blot, W.J., et al. Int. J. Cancer 28:685-689, 1981.
39. Philips, L., and Snowdon, D.A. Cancer Res. 45:2403s-2408s, 1983.
40. Katsouyanni, K., Trichopoulos, D., Boyle, P., et al. Int. J. Cancer 38:815-820, 1086.
41. Lubin, F., Wax, Y., and Modan, B. JNCI. 77:605-612, 1986.
42. Jones, D.Y., Schatzkin, A., Green, S.B., et al. JNCI. 79:465-471, 1987.
43. Willet, W.C., Stampfer, M.J., Colditz, G.A., et al. N. Engl. J. Med. 316:22-28, 1987.
44. Hirohata, T., Nomura, A.M.Y., Hankin, J.H., et al. JNCI. 78:595-600, 1987.
45. Rohan, T.E., McMichael, A.J., Baghurst, P.A. Am. J. Epidemiol. 128:478-489, 1988.
46. Marubini, E., Decarli, A., Costa, A., et al. Cancer 61:173-180, 1988.
47. Hiatt, R.A., and Bawol, R.D. Am. J. Epidemiol. 120:676-683, 1984.
48. O'Connell, D.L., Hulka, B.S., Chambless, L.E., et al. JNCI. 78:229-234, 1987.
49. La Vecchia, C., Decarli, A., Franceschi, S., et al. Am. J. Epidemiol. 120:350-357, 1984.
50. Schatzkin, A., Jones, Y., Hoover, R.N., et al. N. Engl. J. Med. 316:1169-1173, 1987.
51. Willett, W.C., Stampfer, M.J., Colditz, G.A., et al. N. Engl. J. Med. 316:1174-1180, 1987.
52. Harvey, E.B., Schairer, C., Brinton, L.A., et al. JNCI. 78:657-661, 1987.
53. Rosenberg, L., Slone, D., Shapiro, S., et al. Lancet 1:267-271, 1982.
54. Begg, C.B., Walker, A.M., Wessen, B., et al. Lancet 1:293-294, 1983.

18

TOWARDS A BREAST CANCER VACCINE?

C. TOMASETTO, C. GAUTIER, M. HAREUVENI, D.H. WRESCHNER[1],
M.P. KIENY[2], M.C. RIO, P. CHAMBON & R. LATHE

LGME-CNRS & U184-INSERM, 11 Rue Humann, 67085 Strasbourg,
France; [1]Department of Microbiology, Tel Aviv University,
Ramat Aviv, Israel; [2]Transgene S.A., 11 Rue de Molsheim,
67000 Strasbourg, France.

INTRODUCTION

Approximately one woman in 11 develops breast cancer
during her lifetime and mortality can approach 50%: breast
cancer is responsible for one third of all deaths in women
aged between 30 to 50. For this reason much intensive
research has concentrated upon improving existing therapeutic strategies and upon the development of new procedures for the prevention and/or treatment of breast
cancer.

Vaccinia virus (VV), a typical poxvirus used extensively to control and eradicate smallpox, is now widely
used as a live recombinant vector for the expression of
foreign antigens. Inoculation with VV-recombinants expressing structural antigens of viruses or parasites often
leads to the development of protective immunity (reviewed
in 1) and we have previously demonstrated the efficacy of
a VV-recombinant expressing the rabies virus glycoprotein
in conferring protection against rabies (ref. 2 for
review).

We have used a rat model experimental system to explore the possibility of using live VV recombinants in
anti-tumor immunization and we discuss the possibility of
extending this approach to breast cancer.

A RODENT MODEL FOR TUMOR VACCINATION

Polyoma virus (PyV) is a small DNA virus that causes a variety of tumors in rodents. Tumorigenesis involves integration of the PyV genome and transformed cells express three early viral proteins: large-T (LT), middle-T (MT), and small-T (ST). Because the proteins are generated by differential splicing of a common precursor transcript, the ST protein is equivalent to the N-terminal segment of MT. To test whether VV recombinants expressing PyV early proteins might elicit anti-tumor immunity, three recombinant viruses separately expressing the three T proteins were constructed (3); a further recombinant, VV-Cfr, was constructed expressing the isolated C-terminal segment of MT protein.

Fischer rats inoculated with PyV-transformed syngeneic rat cells rapidly develop tumors that kill the host animal. Animals were vaccinated with the VV-T recombinants and challenged by subcutaneous seeding with syngeneic PyV-transformed cells. In Table 1 animals receiving the LT, MT or Cfr recombinants developed small tumors that rapidly regressed. Further, a proportion of animals already bearing tumors could be induced to reject their tumors by inoculation with the appropriate recombinant (3).

More recent experiments have shown that inoculation with purified recombinant ST is capable of inducing PyV anti-tumor immunity (4), demonstrating that a protective epitope lies in the N-terminal (ST) region of the MT protein. In the VV system the ST recombinant VV was ineffective and we have observed stimulated growth of PyV tumors in animals inoculated with the recombinant (unpublished). A VV recombinant expressing the isolated C-terminal MT-Cfr segment was however effective, if not better, than the recombinant expressing intact MT. These results indicate that the identity of the dominant protective epitope may differ according to the means of administration of the antigen. It is of note that none of the PvV proteins appears to be present at the surface of

Table 1. Vaccination against PyV-transformed cells

Vaccine	Tumor rejection	
	Expt. 1	Expt.2
Challenge cells: PYT21		
VV-LT	5/8	nd
VV-MT	14/15	4/4
VV-ST	0/6	nd
VV-Cfr	nd	5/6
Challenge cells: MTT4		
VV-LT	nd	0/6
VV-MT	nd	4/6
VV-Cfr	nd	5/6

Groups of 4-week old female Fisher rats were immunized twice (intradermal) with the purified vaccinia recombinant (10^7 pfu) and challenged by subcutaneous seeding of syngeneic tumor cells expressing the entire PyV genome (PYT21) or the MT protein alone (MTT4) as described (3). nd, not determined.

the transformed cell, demonstrating that an efficient immune response can be directed against internal antigens. Although sera from tumor-bearing animals react exclusively with the shared N-terminal region of the T proteins (not shown), the C-terminal segment of the MT protein is highly effective as an anti-tumor immunogen (above). Antibody--based screening techniques would fail to reveal this epitope, indicating that caution should be observed in the use of immunological procedures designed to identify target antigens and/or epitopes associated with human tumors.

A VIRAL ETIOLOGY FOR BREAST CANCER?

Mammary tumors in mouse are commonly associated with Mouse Mammary Tumor Virus (MMTV) infection. Tumorigenesis involves integration of the MMTV retrovirus genome at specific loci in the mouse genome, and activated ex-

pression of adjacent genes disrupts normal growth control
processes in mammary tissue. In support of a viral etiology for breast cancer, virus particles have been detected
in human milk (5), and retrovirus-like particles have been
found in cultured T47D breast cancer cells (6) or in mono-
cytes from breast cancer patients (7). Further, expression
of an endogenous human retrovirus has been detected in
some breast tumor cell lines (8,9). However, there is as
yet no firm evidence for a viral etiology of human breast
cancer. For this reason we have sought to identify novel
antigens present in breast tumors that may afford targets
for active immunotherapy.

BREAST CANCER ASSOCIATED ANTIGENS

The PS2 protein

PS2 protein is a small (7 kilodalton) secreted protein with structural analogies to a growth factor. Expression of the PS2 gene is estrogen-inducible in the
breast tumor line MCF7 (10) and PS2 is specifically
expressed by approximately 40% of human breast tumors
(11). Although the function of PS2 is unknown, a possible
role as an autocrine growth factor has been discussed
(12).

We have attempted to develop a test system in which
the efficacy of VV recombinants expressing PS2, or sub-
segments of PS2, might be evaluated. Transgenic mice (13)
were constructed specifically expressing PS2 in the lactating mammary gland: the PS2 coding sequence (10,12) was
fused to the control region of the murine whey acidic
protein (WAP) promoter and introduced into the mouse germline. Lactating adult females specifically express the
hybrid WAP-PS2 gene in mammary gland and PS2 protein is
secreted into milk. No pathology was observed in these
animals (or in their suckling young), suggesting that PS2
is not a transforming growth factor for mouse mammary
tissue (unpublished).

Until recently PS2 expression was thought to be
specific to human breast tumors. However, we recently
determined that PS2 is produced by normal human stomach
(14) and anti-PS2 vaccination may thus be contraindicated.

c-erbB2 protein

c-erbB2 (her) encodes a 180 kilodalton cell-surface
protein closely related to the epidermal growth factor
(EGF) receptor and is equivalent to the rat neu oncogene
product (15). However, the molecular ligand for c-erbB2 is
unknown. The gene is amplified and/or overexpressed in a
significant proportion of breast tumor samples (eg. 16-18)
although expression has been observed in other secretory
epithelial tissues (15). We have constructed VV recombinants bearing c-erbB2 coding sequences, however, no expression of the encoded protein has yet been observed
(unpublished). This approach has not been encouraged by
results (19) obtained using VV recombinants expressing the
rat c-erbB2 equivalent, neu. Although rejection of syngeneic tumor cells expressing rat neu was observed in mice
vaccinated with the VV-neu recombinant, no rejection occurred when the recombinant was employed in the cognate rat
model (19). These results may indicate that the rat is
immunologically tolerant to self neu, casting doubts upon
the possibility of productive vaccination against c-erbB2
in man.

The H23 antigen

An alternative target may be afforded by mucin-like
proteins. In a study designed to detect new mammary tumor
specific antigens, Keydar and colleagues (20) prepared
monoclonal antibodies directed against particulate antigens released by T47D mammary tumor cells. Western blotting with one such antibody, H23, identifies a large
variable-sized glycoprotein. Immunohistochemical staining
has revealed that the majority of breast tumors (91%)
express an elevated level of the H23 antigen (H23Ag) in
the cytoplasm. In normal mammary tissue, as well as in
other tissues, H23Ag expression is weak to indetectable

and apical in contrast to cytoplasmic. Cloning of H23Ag coding sequences from the human genome has revealed that a large central segment of the gpH23 gene consists of a multiple tandem repeat of a 60 nucleotide domain encoding a 20 amino acid sequence motif (21, and unpublished data). The available data indicate that H23Ag is very similar to the mucin-like proteins described by other groups (22-25). Repeat elements from the H23Ag gene have been linked to a secretion signal sequence and a transmembrane membrane anchoring domain (in preparation), and the biological properties of a VV recombinant expressing this fusion protein are under examination (unpublished).

DISCUSSION

Vaccinia (VV) recombinants expressing viral or parasite antigens are effective immunogens (1) and we have extended this approach to tumor prevention. VV recombinants expressing early proteins of polyomavirus were constructed, and rats inoculated with VV-polyoma recombinants resisted challenge with syngeneic polyoma-transformed tumor cells (3). Because human breast cancer is not known to have a viral etiology we have sought to identify novel breast-tumor specific antigens that may afford targets for prevention or treatment of breast cancer.

PS2 protein, originally thought to be specific to breast tumors, is now known to be expressed in normal stomach (14). Although anti-PS2 immunotherapy may be contraindicated for this reason, it remains an open question whether immune damage of the stomach epithelium may occur and, if so, whether this might be an acceptable penalty in the prevention of breast tumor metastasis. The cell-surface receptor encoded by the c-erbB2 gene affords an alternative target. However, experiments with VV recombinants expressing the rat c-erbB2 equivalent, neu, indicate that the animal may be immunologically tolerant to this antigen (19). A third antigen, H23Ag, is detected in the majority of breast tumor biopsy samples (20).

However, low levels of this antigen can also detected in normal breast tissue and anti-H23Ag vaccination may be restricted to the prevention of metastasis following mastectomy. Because none of the three antigens examined appears entirely suitable as a vaccine target the search for new breast cancer specific antigens must continue.

ACKNOWLEGEMENTS
      This work was supported by a project grant from the Federation Nationale des Centres de Lutte Contre le Cancer, the INSERM (CNAMTS grant), the Association pour la Recherche sur le Cancer, and the Fondation pour la Recherche Médicale. M.H. and D.H.W. are recipients of EMBO fellowships. We thank E. Lucassen, A.C. Andres, and N. Hynes for providing the c-erbB2 coding sequence.

REFERENCES
1. Moss, B. and Flexner, C. Ann. Rev. Immunol. 5: 305-324,1987.
2. Wiktor, T.J., Kieny, M.P. and Lathe, R. Appl. Virol. Res. 1: 69-90, 1988.
3. Lathe, R., Kieny, M.P., Gerlinger, P., Clertant, P., Guizani, I., Cuzin, F. & Chambon, P. Nature 326: 878-880, 1987.
4. Ramqvist, T., Pallas, D.O., DeAnda, J., Ahrlund-Richter, L., Reinholdsson, G., Roberts, T.M., Schaffhausen, B. and Dalianis, T. Intl. J. Cancer 42: 123-128, 1988.
5. Moore, D.H., Charney, J., Kramarsky, B., Lasfargues, E.Y., Sarkar, N.H., Brennan, M., Burrows, J.H., Sirsat, S.M., Paymaster, J.C. and Vaidya, A.B. Nature 229: 611-615, 1971.
6. Keydar, I., Ohno, T., Nayak, R., Sweet, R., Simoni, F., Weiss, F., Karby, S., Mesa-Tejada, R. and Spiegelman, S. Proc. Natl. Acad. Sci. USA 81: 4188-4192, 1984.
7. Al-Sumidaie, A.M., Leinster, S.J., Hart, C.A., Green, C.D. and McCarthy, K. Lancet 2/9: 5-9, 1988.
8. Ono, M., Kawakami, M. and Ushikubo, H. J. Virol. 61: 2059- 2062, 1987.
9. Franklin, G.C., Chretien, S., Hanson, I.M., Rochefort, H., May, F.E.B. and Westley, B.R. J. Virol. 62: 1203-

1210, 1988.

10. Masiokowski, P., Breathnach, R., Bloch, J., Gannon, F., Krust, A. and Chambon, P. Nucl. Acids Res. 10: 7895-7903, 1982.

11. Rio, M.C., Bellocq, J.P., Gairard, B., Rasmussen, U.B., Krust, A., Koehl, C., Calderoli, H., Schiff, V., Renaud, R. and Chambon, P. Proc. Natl. Acad. Sci. USA 84: 9243-9247, 1987.

12. Jakowlew, S.B., Breathnach, R., Jeltsch, J.M., Masiakowsky, P. and Chambon, P. Nucl. Acids Res. 12, 2861-2878, 1984.

13. Palmiter, R.D. and Brinster, R.L. Ann. Rev. Genet. 20: 465-499, 1986.

14. Rio, M.C., Belloca, J.P., Daniel, J.Y., Tomasetto, C., Lathe, R., Chanard, M.P., Batzenschlager, A. and Chambon, P. Science 241: 705-708; 1988.

15. Kokai, Y., Cohen, J.A., Drebin, J.A. and Greene, M.I. Proc. Natl. Acad. Sci. USA 84: 8498-8501, 1987.

16. Slamon, D.J., Clark, G.M., Wong, S.G., Ullrich, A. and McGuire, W.L. Science 235: 177-182, 1987.

17. Berger, M.S., Locher, G.W., Saurer, S., Gullick, W.J., Waterfield, M.D., Groner, B. and Hynes, N. Cancer Res. 48: 1238-1243, 1988.

18. Tal, M., Wetzler, M., Josefberg, Z., Deutch, A., Gutman, M., Assaf, D., Kris, R., Shiloh, Y., Givol, D. and Schlessinger, J. Cancer Res. 48: 1517-1520, 1988.

19. Bernards, R., Destree, A., McKenzie, S., Gordon, E., Weinberg, R.A. and Panicali, D. Proc. Natl. Acad. Sci. USA 84: 6854-6858, 1987.

20. Keydar, I., Chou, C.S., Hareuveni, M., Tsarfaty, I., Sahar, E., Chaitchik, S. and Hizi, A. Proc. Natl. Acad. Sci., in press, 1989.

21. Hareuveni, M., Tsarfaty, I., Weiss, M., Keydar, I. and Wreschner, D.H. Submitted, 1989.

22. Swallow, D.M., Gendler, S., Griffiths, B., Corney, G., Taylor-Papadimitriou, J. and Bramwell, M.E. Nature 328: 82-84, 1987.

23. Gendler, S.J., Burchell, J.M., Duhig, T., Lamport, D., White, R., Parker, M. and Taylor-Papadimitriou, J. Proc. Natl. Acad. Sci. USA 84: 6060-6064, 1987.

24. Siddiqui, J., Abe, M., Hayes, D., Shani, E., Yunis, E. and Kufe, D. Proc. Natl. Acad. Sci. USA 85: 2320-2323, 1988.

25. Mesa-Tejada, R., Palakodety, R.B., Leon, J.A., Khatcherian, A.O. and Greaton, C.J. Amer. J. Path. 130: 305-314, 1988.

19

BREAST TUMOR CELL HETEROGENEITY AND EVOLUTION IN
RESPONSE TO MONOCLONAL ANTIBODY THERAPY

J.A. PETERSON, E.W. BLANK, M.A. WONG, J.S. PENG,
R. CAILLEAU and R.L. CERIANI

John Muir Cancer and Aging Research Institute,
2055 N. Broadway, Walnut Creek, CA   94596

INTRODUCTION

One aspect of the biology of breast cancer that
hinders cure is tumor cell heterogeneity and
phenotypic variability. Some tumor cells may be
killed by the therapy, but the ability of a tumor
cell population to adapt to a hostile environment
invariably results in progression of the disease.
Either the tumor cells are already resistant to the
therapeutic drug or develop resistance during the
course of the treatment. New prospects for breast
cancer therapy have arisen with the development of
monoclonal antibodies (1,2), but here again cell
heterogeneity in the expression of the target antigen
must be overcome. One advantage of MoAb therapy over
other types of therapy is that the target antigen can
be clearly identified, specifically selected for
therapy, and its expression studied. Also, the MoAb
can be tailored for therapy, designed for efficient
conjugation to cytotoxic drugs, and/or modified to
reduce immunogenicity or for better clearance from
circulation.

In order to understand the relationship between
target antigen expression and the effectiveness of
MoAb therapy we have analyzed quantitatively, using
flow cytometry, the expression of two different
epitopes of a large molecular weight breast mucin (3)
in different human breast carcinomas transplanted in

nude mice that are treated with radioiodinated MoAb.
The ultimate goal is to establish criteria for
selecting MoAbs, selecting patients, predicting
responsiveness, evaluating outcome, and understanding
the reasons for non-responsiveness. It would be
expected that several other factors would influence
effectiveness of MoAb therapy, such as growth rate of
the tumor cells, vascularization, penetration of the
therapeutic MoAb, radiation resistance of the
particular tumor cells, and host susceptibility to
radiation, but target antigen concentration and tumor
cell heterogeneity and distribution in the tumor seem
to be two of the critical factors to consider. The
MoAbs used in this study, that were prepared using
the human milk fat globule membrane as an immunogen,
identify different epitopes on a large molecular
weight mucin (3) that is present on the surface of
normal breast epithelial cells, primarily the apical
surface facing the lumen, while in breast carcinomas
it is often expressed at higher levels than on the
normal cells and appears both on the cell surface and
in the cytoplasm. For this study we have developed
methods, using a flow cytometer, to measure
quantitatively the antigen content both on the cell
surface and in the cytoplasm. The antigen content,
distribution, and variability was evaluated before
and after therapy in order to assess the effect of
radiolabeled MoAb therapy on the target antigen
expression.

MATERIALS AND METHODS
Flow Cytometry

Single cell suspensions of breast carcinoma cells
were analyzed on a Coulter EPICS 753 flow cytometer.
The preparation of single cell suspensions of
cultured cells has been described previously (4).

Briefly, the cells in monolayer culture were removed
from the culture vessel with trypsin, then suspended
in medium containing methyl cellulose, layered over
agar, and cultured for 48 hours (4). Tumors
transplanted in nude mice were removed from the mice
and mechanically dispersed. The single cell
suspensions were stained with fluoresceinated MoAbs,
Mc5 and BrE1. The MoAbs were fluoresceinated by the
method of Kearney and Lawton (5). All staining with
the fluoresceinated MoAb was carried out at 4° C.
Surface antigen content was represented by staining
of viable unfixed cells while total antigen content
(surface and cytoplasm) was obtained by staining
cells that had been fixed in 70% ethanol in PBS for
30 minutes. In all cases, data from at least 20,000
cells were collected. The flow cytometer histograms
were analyzed by the Coulter IMMUNO program using as
a control histogram the same cells stained with a
fluoresceinated non-specific IgG_1 (Coulter
Immunology, Hialeah, FL) to determine the relative
mean fluorescence of the positive cells, the
percentage positive cells, and the coefficient of
variation. Flow cytometer data was collected both on
logarithmic and linear scales, since the latter
allowed determination of the coefficient of
variation. In order to compare the mean fluorescence
intensity of different samples run on different days
the fluoresceinated MoAbs were standardized using
SIMPLY CELLULAR® beads (Flow Cytometry Standards
Corp., North Carolina), and then antigen content is
expressed as relative mean channel number which is
proportional to the relative mean number of antibody
molecules bound per cell.

Experimental radiolabeled MoAb therapy

Breast carcinoma cell lines were maintained in
culture as previously described (4), or as

transplantable tumors in immunodeficient BALB/c nu/nu
nude mice. The 3 cell lines with prefix MDA-MB are
part of a collection of 19 breast cell lines (6) that
we are in the process of adapting to growth in nude
mice. In the therapy experiments, quadruplicate mice
were treated with a single dose of 500 microcuries of
^{131}I-labeled MoAb approximately two weeks after
transplantation when the tumors were well
vascularized and about 100 mm^3 in volume.
Therapeutic effectiveness was determined at 15 days
after injection by comparison with increase in size
of tumors in comparable control untreated mice, and
expressed as percentage inhibition of growth (%IG)
(7). Tumors that re-initiated growth were allowed to
grow for about 5 weeks more before being excised for
flow cytometry analysis for antigen content. Tumors
from untreated mice that were transplanted at the
same time were used as controls.

RESULTS

We have systematically studied surface and
cytoplasmic content of two different epitopes of the
breast mucin, identified by MoAbs Mc5 and BrE1,
respectively, in a collection of different breast
carcinoma cell lines that we have also adapted for
growth as transplanted tumors in nude mice. As can
be seen in Table 1, each of the 8 breast carcinoma
cell lines is different with regard to the level of
expression of the two epitopes, the percentage of
positive cells, and also the ratio of surface to
cytoplasmic expression. In general, Mc5 usually
stains the cell surface, while BrE1 often stains
primarily the cytoplasm. However, there are
exceptions; for example, the Mc5 epitope is expressed
primarily on cell surface of MDA-MB-331 cells, while
in the MDA-MB-361 cell line, it is expressed almost

Table 1. Comparison of surface and cytoplasmic binding of Mc5 and BrE-1 to different breast carcinoma cell lines measured by flow cytometry.

Cell Line	Surface Antigen				Total Antigen (Surf. & Cyto.)			
	% Positive		Relative Mean Channel #		% Positive		Relative Mean Channel #	
	Mc5	BrE-1	Mc5	BrE-1	Mc5	BrE-1	Mc5	BrE-1
SKBR3	65%	4%	214	0	96%	85%	690	122
ZR-75	84%	44%	3606	326	91%	91%	2201	679
MDA-MB-361	1%	0%	741	430	99%	98%	321	104
MDA-MB-331	96%	13%	2069	76	97%	64%	2324	201
MCF-7	91%	8%	1338	185	93%	99%	2016	130
T47D	61%	4%	53	27	97%	95%	111	135
MDA-MB-435	3%	1%	85	77	99%	99%	23	33
MX1	37%	96%	74	187	98%	99%	177	304

excusively in the cytoplasm (Figure 1). For the MX1
breast tumor, Mc5 stains more in the cytoplasm than
on the cell surface, while BrE1 stains 96% of the
cells on the surface. For both Mc5 and BrE1, there
can be a 50- to 100-fold variation from one tumor to
another in mean epitope concentration (both surface
and cytoplasmic), although a higher level of
expression of one epitope does not mean a high
expression of the other. Since we have recently
isolated lambda gt11 cDNA clones that express fusion
proteins that are recognized by both Mc5 and BrE1
(unpublished results), we can clearly state that
their epitopes are at least partially polypeptide and
on the same molecule. Therefore, the differences in
expression of the two different epitopes is probably
partly due to different processing of the molecule
which allow exposure or masking of the different
epitopes. In this respect it should be noted (Table
1) that for most of the breast tumors, even when a
small percentage of the cells had surface staining,
virtually all the cells have some of this high
molecular weight mucin antigen, be it in the
cytoplasm or on the membrane.

In order to study the effect of MoAb therapy on
target antigen content, we treated nude mice carrying
different breast carcinomas with single doses of
^{131}I-labeled Mc5. The mice were treated at least
two weeks after transplanting, when the tumors were
about 100 mm^3, vascularized, and well established.
Four different breast carcinomas were studied that
differed significantly in target antigen content
(Table 2). With each of the different breast tumors
there was a significance response to the
radioimmunotherapy, although the therapeutic
effectiveness, expressed as percentage inhibition

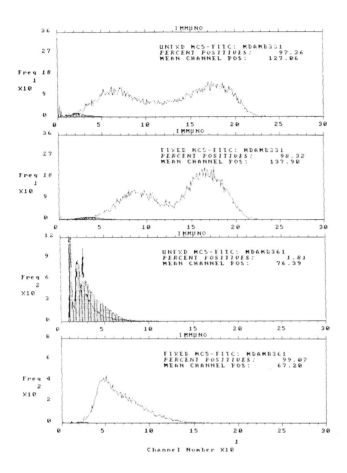

Fig. 1. Flow cytometry analysis of surface and
cytoplasmic expression of an epitope on a large
molecular weight breast mucin identified by MoAb Mc5
in two different breast carcinoma cell lines,
MDA-MB-331 and MDA-MB-361. Staining of unfixed
(UNFXD) cells represents surface antigen and staining
of fixed cells (FIXED) represents total antigen
(surface and cytoplasm). The abscissa, representing
relative fluorescence (channel number), is a
logarithmic scale, with the open histogram being
Mc5-FITC stained cells and the shaded histogram being
control IgG_1-FITC stained cells. Percentage
positive cells and mean channel number of positive
cells is obtained by Coulter IMMUNO analysis program.

Table 2. Effect of 131I-labeled MoAb treatment of immunodeficient nude mice carrying different human breast carcinomas on target antigen content measured by flow cytometry.

TUMOR	%IG 15 days[1]	Percent Positive	Mean Antigen Content[3]	Antigen Content Index
MDA-MB-435	64%			
Untreated (01)[2]		23%	75	17
Untreated (02)		13%	69	9
Treated (03)		38%	81	30
Treated (04)		28%	102	28
MDA-MB-331	47%			
Untreated (05)		20%	253	50
Treated (06)		65%	413	268
MCF-7	22%			
Untreated (07)		19%	357	67
Treated (08)		42%	256	107
MX1	97%			
Untreated (09)		90%	167	150
Untreated (10)		59%	217	128
Treated (11)		77%	452	348
Treated (12)		94%	496	466

1 %IG - 15 days = Percentage inhibition of growth 15 days after beginning treatment.
2 Mouse identification number.
3 Relative channel number (see Materials and Methods).

of growth (%IG) (See Materials and Methods) 15 days after treatment, varied from 22% to 97% (Table 2).

After the initial destruction of the tumors by radioimmunotherapy with ^{131}I-labeled Mc5, the mice were left for several weeks to allow the tumors to re-grow, then the tumors were removed, the tumor cells dispersed and analyzed on the flow cytometer for target antigen content with Mc5 (Table 2). The most important result from these studies was that in no case was there any reduction in the target antigen content in the surviving tumor cell population nor in the percentage of positive cells. In contrast, for all four different breast tumors there was a significant increase in either the mean antigen content or percentage positive cells or both (Table 2.) In order to combine percentage positive cells and mean antigen content, we derive what we refer to as Antigen Content Index, which is the product of the two. With all four tumors there was a 2- to 4-fold increase in the Antigen Content Index after radioimmunotherapy with Mc5. These results were unexpected and clearly different from previous results with treatment of breast tumors in nude mice with a cocktail of native unconjugated MoAbs, where there was a significant decrease in antigen level in tumors that grew in the treated mice compared to untreated mice (1).

DISCUSSION

The advantage of flow cytometry for measuring antigen expression in breast tumor cell populations is that it can give a detailed picture of the antigen distribution in a heterogeneous tumor cell population. This picture includes; the mean antigen content per cell, the percentage of positive cells, distribution of antigen levels among the positive cells, and also detect subpopulations within the positive cells. In addition, by staining both viable and fixed cells we are able to obtain values for both surface antigen content and total antigen content (surface plus cytoplasmic). Furthermore, by standardizing the fluorescent labeled MoAbs with SIMPLY CELLULAR® beads, we are able to determine the actual number of MoAb molecules bound per cell (although in these studies we only express them as relative channel number).

One conclusion from these studies of the expression of two different epitopes on the large molecular weight breast mucin glycoprotein in 8 different breast carcinoma cell lines, is that there is not only a single cell heterogeneity in expression of these different epitopes within a tumor cell population, but also a tremendous difference from one breast tumor to another, both with regard to total antigen content and intracellular distribution. Some of this quantitative variations can be due to different levels of expression of the mucin antigen, but they must also be due to differences in processing of the molecule, e.g. degree of glycosylation that would mask or hinder MoAb access to its epitope. In addition, the rate at which the antigens are released from the breast tumor cells would also effect the level of cellular antigen measured by flow cytometry, since breast tumor cells do release these breast mucin antigens into circulation both in nude mice (8) and in breast cancer patients (9). Another conclusion from the studies using two different MoAbs against the breast mucin and looking at both surface and cytoplasmic content of the epitopes, is that nearly every tumor

cell in the population, if not all, have this large
molecular weight mucin, although there is
considerable variation in the level of expression of
different epitopes. Since the function of this large
molecular weight breast mucin is not yet understood,
we do not know the biological impact of this vast
variation in expression of different epitopes of the
molecule. However, from a practical point of view
the adaptation of different breast tumors (15 of them
to date) to grow in nude mice, each with different
and distinct phenotypic characteristics, provides us
a system to evaluate the relationships between target
antigen content and MoAb therapy.

The present results do not show any clear
relationship between the original antigen content of
the breast tumor and therapeutic effectiveness,
although 4 different tumors is not sufficient to make
a definite conclusion. We do know from previous
experiments, that non-breast tumors with no target
antigen are not responsive to this treatment (2).
Other factors must also play a role in responsive,
such as tumor growth rate, as could be the case for
MCF-7 tumor which has a high target antigen content
but also grows much slower than MX1, which is very
responsiveness. The relative responsiveness of the
MDA-MB-435 tumor compared to MCF-7 tumor, in spite of
having several fold less antigen than MCF-7, could
suggest that there may be a relatively low threshold
in target antigen content above which
radioimmunotherapy can be effective. In other words,
since radiolabelled MoAb does not have to bind to
each individual tumor cell to kill it, and since
cells will be killed in a surrounding area depending
on the energy of the particular radioisotope, there
need be only a sufficient percentage of antigen

containing tumor cells, or sufficient antigen in the vicinity of the tumor (i.e., released antigen) to allow homing of enough therapeutic MoAb. This critical level is important to know when evaluating the antigen content in a patient's tumor and deciding whether or not to try radioimmunotherapy.

The most important result from these studies of the effect of radioiodinated MoAb therapy on target antigen content in the treated tumors is that there is no selection for a reduced antigen content in the surviving tumor cell population. Surprisingly, there is an increase in antigen content as a result of the treatment. This increase occurred with four different transplantable breast tumors, so it appears to be a general phenomenon; although, there was not always an increase in every individual mouse. An explanation for this increase is that the radiolabeled Mc5 kills preferentially dividing cells due to the ionizing radiation and not neccesarily those cells that have a high antigen content. It is possible that more differentiated cells with a higher antigen content may be less likely dividing and thus selectively survive the irradiation of the treatment. This result is extremely important with regard to prospects for repeated fractionated treatment of breast cancer patients. From current knowledge on the clinical course of breast cancer, it is apparent that if radiolabeled MoAbs are going to be effective in curing breast cancer or increasing survival significantly, repeated courses of treatment will be necessary. The present results mean that repeated targeting of the tumor will be possible. Therefore, designing of chimeric human-mouse MoAbs in order to evade the immune response of the patient that will allow such repeated treatments appears to be a rational approach.

This work is supported by NIH grants RO1 CA39936, RO1 CA39932, PO1 CA42767, and BRSG RRO5929.

REFERENCES

1. Ceriani, R.L., Blank, E.W. and Peterson, J.A. Cancer Res. <u>47</u>: 532-540, 1987.
2. Ceriani, R.L. and Blank, E.W. Cancer Res. <u>48</u>: 4664-4672, 1988.
3. Ceriani, R.L., Peterson, J.A., Lee, J.Y., Moncada, R. and Blank, E.W. Cell Genetics <u>9</u>: 45-427, 1983.
4. Peterson, J.A., Bartholomew, J.C., Stampfer, M. and Ceriani, R.L. Exp. Cell Biol. <u>49</u>: 1-14, 1981.
5. Kearney, J.F. and Lawton, A.R. J. Immuno. <u>115</u>: 671-676, 1975.
6. Cailleau, R., Olivé, M. and Cruciger, Q.J. In Vitro <u>14</u>: 911-915, 1978.
7. Ceriani, R.L., Battifora, H., Blank, E.W., Peterson, J.A. and Zoellner, C. <u>In</u>: Breast Cancer Immunodiagnosis and Immunotherapy, (Ed. Ceriani, R.L.), Plenum Publishing, New York, in Press, 1989.
8. Sasaki, M., Peterson, J.A., Wara, W. and Ceriani, R.L. Cancer <u>4</u>: 2204-2210, 1981.
9. Ceriani, R.L., Sasaki, M., Sussman, H., Wara, W.M. and Blank E.W. Proc. Natl. Acad. Sci. USA <u>79</u>: 5420-5424, 1982.

INDEX